CW01208998

RE-
DISCOVERED

RE-DISCOVERED

Down & Dirty Spirituality to revitalise who you really are, where you're going and what you came here to do!

Sharon Eden

First published in 2024 by Intellectual Perspective Press
© Copyright Sharon Eden

All rights reserved. No part of this publication may be reproduced, stored in or introduced into a retrieval system, or transmitted, in any form, or by any means (electronic, mechanical, photocopying, recording or otherwise) without the prior written permission of the publisher.

The right of Sharon Eden to be identified as the author of this work has been asserted in accordance with the Copyright, Designs and Patents Act 1988.

This book is sold subject to the condition that it shall not, by way of trade or otherwise, be lent, resold, hired out, or otherwise circulated without the publisher's prior consent in any form of binding or cover other than that in which it is published and without a similar condition including this condition being imposed on the subsequent purchaser.

The purpose of this book is to educate and entertain. The author and Intellectual Perspective Press shall have neither liability nor responsibility to any person or entity with respect to any loss or damage caused, or alleged to have been caused, directly or indirectly, by the information contained in this book.

Book Interior and E-book Design by Amit Dey
(amitdey2528@gmail.com)

To find out more about our authors and books visit:
www.intellectualperspective.com

"Not until we are lost do we begin
to understand ourselves"

Henry David Thoreau

"As you start to walk on the way,
the way appears."

Jalāl al-Dīn Muḥammad Rūmī

TABLE OF CONTENTS

Praise for RE-DISCOVERED xi

Foreword xiii

Sarah xvii

To begin… xxi

The Treasure Map ....**xxv**

    The Treasure Map brief location key… xxix

1 DOWN & DIRTY SPIRITUALITY **1**

    What spirituality is and isn't… 3

    What's Down & Dirty Spirituality? 9

    Imagination and a resource for your adventure 17

2 WHO ARE YOU? **25**

    Your personality 27

    You are more than your personality 37

    Your connection with the Divine 47

3 WHERE ARE YOU GOING? **53**

    Where have you come from? 57

Where are you going?.................................. 63

Where might you trip yourself up?.................... 69

Where is the resource to overcome your "trip up"?... 75

4 WHAT DID YOU COME HERE TO DO?..............83

Your mission on Earth, purpose, and meaning...... 85

Your spiritual fingerprint............................ 93

Your mission on Earth, purpose, and meaning revisited 99

5 THE END 105

Choice or no choice 107

Evolution and the shape of it........................ 111

Reincarnation but not as you know it! 117

What's next? 121

6 THE END... HONESTLY! 123

The last word.. 127

The Treasure Map Key............................... 131

Biography 141

Acknowledgements 145

More Praise for Re-discovered 149

PRAISE FOR RE-DISCOVERED

Sometimes we need to fall apart so we can have a breakthrough, be reborn and reconstituted. Sharon shows you how to let grace re-form you into a truer, wilder, and more powerful version of who you have always been in essence.

Nick Williams, Leadership Guide,
Speaker and Author of nineteen books including
"The Work We Were Born To Do"

With the tools, stories, and enormous empathy for the moments in life when we are tested, Sharon has produced a powerful book that we can all benefit from reading. A must-read in these changing times when personal understanding and commitment to our own path is critical to our happiness and peace.

Contented, at peace and transformed, what a journey within this book. Throw yourself in and rejuvenate.

Penny Power OBE, CEO, Community Founder,
Author of "Business is Personal"

Down-to-earth and immensely readable, we are led through the major existential questions of identity. Who am I? What is life calling me to do or be? What are the values that I live by? I especially liked the humour and practical approach, allowing us to reframe the edges and challenges that women deal with throughout their lives.

Diana Whitmore, Co-CEO of Growing2gether, Founder of
the Psychosynthesis Trust, Trainer, Coach and Supervisor
in Transpersonal Psychology, Author of "Psychosynthesis
Counselling in Action"

A treasure trove of exercises, insights, and tips, interwoven with Sharon Eden's own story, to help you gain self-awareness. Rather than there being specific "right answers," she skilfully guides you to find the ones that are right for you.

Dorothy Dalton, Founder,
3Plus International Business Services Consultancy

Sharon approaches this subject not only with great gusto but also with humour and sincerity. She has taken some deep psychological concepts and made them easily digestible for the reader as well as offering some great practical tips and exercises to expand the reader's experience.

Judith Firman, Co Author of "Willing to Love - Stories of the Couple's Journey as a Path of Transformation"

I am always sceptical about self-help tomes but this one is authentic, taking us through a journey of Sharon's sometimes painful path to self-discovery. She is there to guide us throughout to the choices on offer and what the right choice for each one of us can be.

Lady Val Corbett, Founder of Lady Val's Professional Network for Women

Wow, what a read! This inspirational and informative book is a must for anyone seeking to reconnect with their inner purpose and embrace a more fulfilling life.

Aruna Rao,
Founder & CEO of Busy Women Networking

FOREWORD

As you are holding this book, I am guessing that you are looking for a timely intervention, a chance to break free from the cycle of dissatisfaction, frustration, feeling lost and disconnected from yourself and the opportunity to step into a life filled with clarity and joy. This book is a gift that helps you revitalise who you really are, where you're going and what you came here to do.

It is a beacon of hope and a roadmap designed to help you navigate the complexities of modern life and rediscover your true self.

Reading RE-DISCOVERED was like witnessing my own life journey on the pages. There were many times in my life when I felt like giving up. The struggle of leaving my ex-husband and becoming a single parent to two boys left me feeling lost and overwhelmed. I faced immense societal pressure and struggled to find direction and financial stability.

During this challenging period, I discovered principles similar to those Sharon shares in her book. By applying these strategies, I reclaimed my sense of purpose and direction.

The transformation wasn't easy or immediate, but it was profound. Sharon's road map in RE-DISCOVERED would have made my journey of rediscovery quicker and easier.

As you turn the pages of this book, prepare to embark on an adventure that will challenge you, inspire you, and ultimately lead you to a place of greater understanding and fulfilment. The journey ahead is one of introspection, discovery, and empowerment. Each chapter is crafted to guide you through a process of transformation, helping you to reconnect with your inner self and unlock the potential that lies within.

I've been blessed to know Sharon for over fifteen years and have always felt and witnessed her passion to help women uncover their true potential and lead lives that are not only successful but deeply meaningful.

The work that Sharon does and the results her clients experience is a testament to the transformative power of self-discovery and personal growth. With her years of experience and countless success stories, I am confident that the insights and strategies shared in RE-DISCOVERED will provide you with the tools you need to overcome your challenges and thrive.

Whether your life mirrors Sarah's experiences, the exemplar in the book, closely or you find similarities in your own journey, RE-DISCOVERED is designed for you. It speaks to the part of you that longs for more, that seeks answers to the existential questions that keep you awake at night.

The answers you seek are within reach, and this book is your companion on the path to a more contented and purposeful life. Welcome to the beginning of your new adventure.

Jacqueline Y B Rogers
Creator of The Athena Network

SARAH

Sarah is a bright articulate 46-year-old professional/businesswoman who's done some personal development and loves reading, self-help books included. She's not religious in the conventional meaning of the word, but has a sense of "something" more.

She has a material life that an outsider would judge as good: comfortable home, a car, and one or two holidays a year. She doesn't feel the need to follow fashion, but likes to dress well in her own style.

She enjoys an occasional visit to the theatre and the Royal Academy. She also loves meeting friends for dinner and the occasional afternoon tea in town.

Lately, she's felt unsettled and restless inside. Sometimes it's even more like nervousness: a tinge of anxiety.

It feels like having the tip-of-the-tongue phenomenon in her physical and sensory being. Like she's just not "getting" something important but she doesn't know what.

Sarah's GP has suggested it might be down to the perimenopause but she's not convinced.

Despite her "good life", she's feeling discontented and, at times, lost and a bit guilty because she's got a comfortable life compared to some others.

Sometimes she potters around, starting a project, then leaving it to start something else without completing either. Like she just can't settle whatever she does.

Sarah does a good cover-up job at work where she can identify with her role, be "work" her and "forget" herself. In fact, it's a blessed relief from the uncertainty she's experiencing.

She also does a cover-up for her logically minded partner, fearing they won't understand, or, if they did, they'd want to "fix" it. She knows it isn't something you can "fix" in that got to DO something about it way.

Indeed, she'd thought a recent holiday was what she needed to get rid of those feelings. Although she'd had a lovely time, there were a couple of occasions, once watching the sunset and once visiting a beautiful island, when she just started to cry and didn't know why.

However, Sarah realised the holiday had just been a distraction, because, once she was back, the discontent and discomfort returned with a vengeance.

That's the trouble with it. Even if it goes away for a while, whatever she does, it always comes back again.

Although her friends and family are lovely, she's begun to question where she actually fits. Sometimes she's experienced herself just observing them socially and not being engaged in what's going on. Like an outsider looking in.

And now, worst of all, she's found herself waking early in the morning and not getting back to sleep easily. She lies still staring into the dark and, worryingly at those times, she's begun to think and feel a bit desperate.

Sometimes she cries quietly so as not to disturb. And, often now, she wakes with thoughts of, "Is this it?", "Is this all my life's ever going to be?" and "There HAS to be more to life than this!"

What that is she has no idea. She also has no idea about what's happening to her.

"Am I going bonkers?" she wonders half-jokingly and half-scared.

Now, you and your life might be a lot like Sarah and hers, a little like Sarah and hers, or not at all. But if anything in Sarah's story strikes a chord, RE-DISCOVERED is definitely for you.

TO BEGIN...

I'd had periods of discontent, restlessness and thoughts like Sarah's from my late twenties, and always found a way forward that was enough to settle them down for a while. Then they would reassert themselves.

It wasn't until I had a breakdown in my forties that I began to sit up and notice the powerful evolutionary push of my Wild Soul. And its inner wisdom urging me to manifest more of who I was designed to be and more of my magnificence.

It's a freakin' hard way to get conscious that I wouldn't recommend.

It's hell on wheels, a total dissolution of who you thought you were and where you thought you were going, accompanied by high anxiety, even terror, and the loss of your everyday life as you'd known it.

If you've already experienced that, my heart goes out to you.

Breaking down to break through is one hell of a gig!

RE-DISCOVERED will help you find a gentler way to rediscover and express the woman you were designed to be, where you're going, and what you came here to do.

And if you haven't experienced a breakdown, great!

RE-DISCOVERED will also help you to rediscover and express more of the woman you were designed to be, where you're going, and what you came here to do.

In fact, magnificent woman, **this is the beginning of an adventure to rediscover and express more of your delicious magnificence and Divine splendour.**

It's not unusual to feel discontented, frustrated or lost at different times in your life for it's rarely a one-and-done cure-all.

So RE-DISCOVERED gives you tools you can use repeatedly as you grow through the meta-adventure that is your life.

I encourage you to think of this time as a rite of passage.

Like a snake shedding its skin because it's become too tight for its growing body, you leave behind some of what's too small for you as you move into a more revitalised and refined you.

In that respect, I encourage you to keep a record of your adventure and I'd suggest you do that through journaling. I don't mean a "Dear Diary" kind of record but a mindful recording of experiences, thoughts, feelings, insights, and ideas.

Think of it as a conversation with yourself, writing about what strikes you, your insights, memories, changes, anything but anything that happens with you as you travel through RE-DISCOVERED.

The founder of Psychosynthesis, Roberto Assagioli, called writing a journal putting "spiritual money into the bank".

Entries in your journal are the deposits. Then, even years later, when something similar occurs, you can find the relevant original deposit and withdraw the insights and techniques you need; taking "spiritual money out of the bank!"

Be aware your experiences, thoughts, feelings, insights, and ideas might not be what you expect and might even seem bizarre or nonsensical to your logical mind. More of that when you get to "Imagination and a resource for your adventure".

Be curious. Take what information you get in whatever form it comes, and all will be revealed.

Having worked professionally with thousands of women over forty years, I know no formulaic quick fix works, even though you might love to have one.

A quick fix might bring initial relief but it soon wears off and you'll find yourself back at square one.

Similarly, I have no easy platitudinal answers. I can't tell you who you are, except generically, and certainly can't tell you where you're going or what you came here to do.

That's information contained in your original design held by your Wild Soul.

You've always had an unconscious "knowing" about this information. What RE-DISCOVERED can do is to stimulate that "knowing" so you become more aware of it.

You'll rediscover more of who you really are, where you're going, and what you came here to do as you go through RE-DISCOVERED page by page.

PS I often mention the Divine. This refers to any benevolent and loving energy you believe is "more than" and resides in what I call "the beyond-beyond". The Universe, Goddess, God… or whatever your name is for it.

AND…

This is not the truth!

As with all of RE-DISCOVERED, take what works for you and leave the rest.

You are allowed!

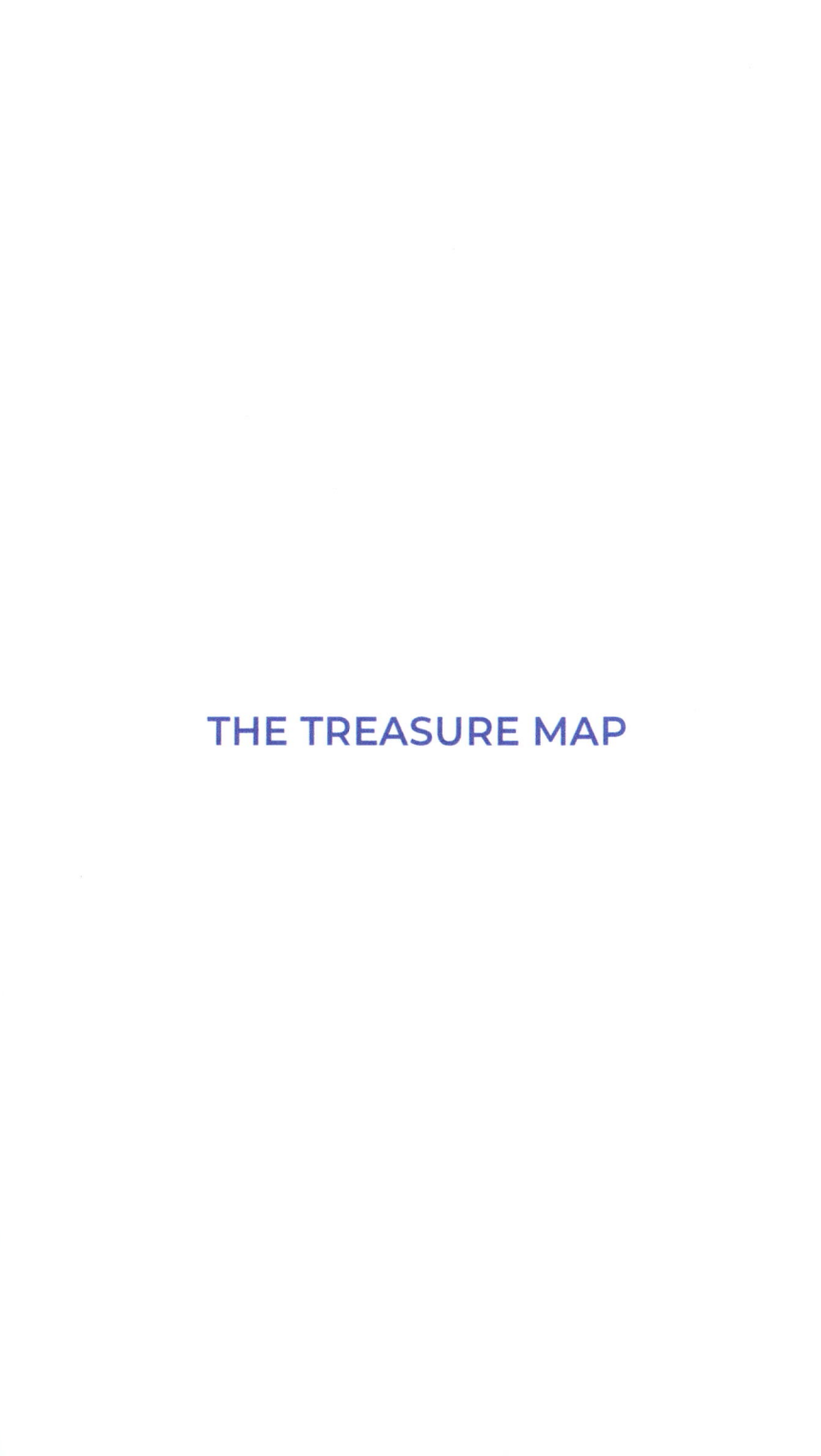

THE TREASURE MAP

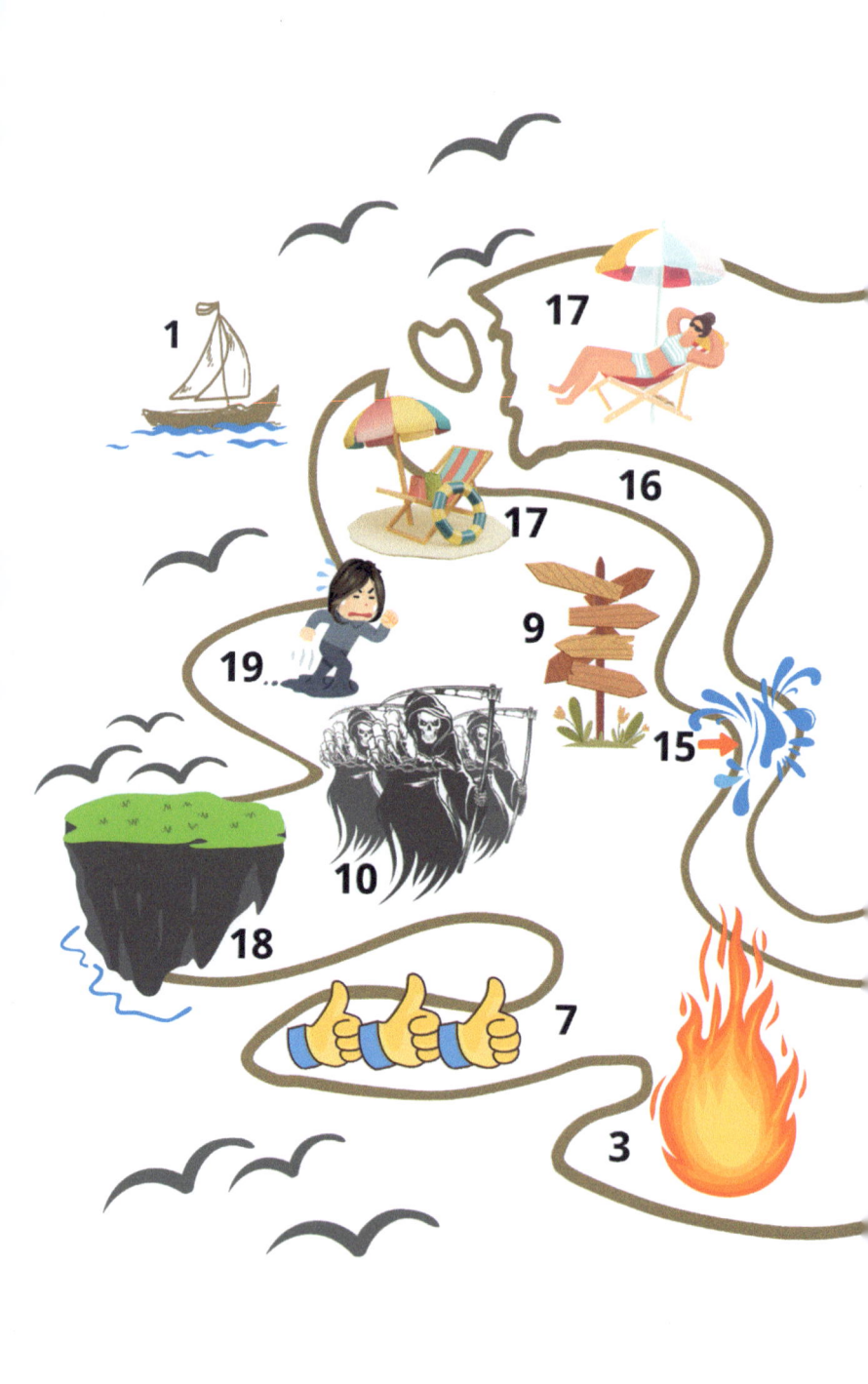

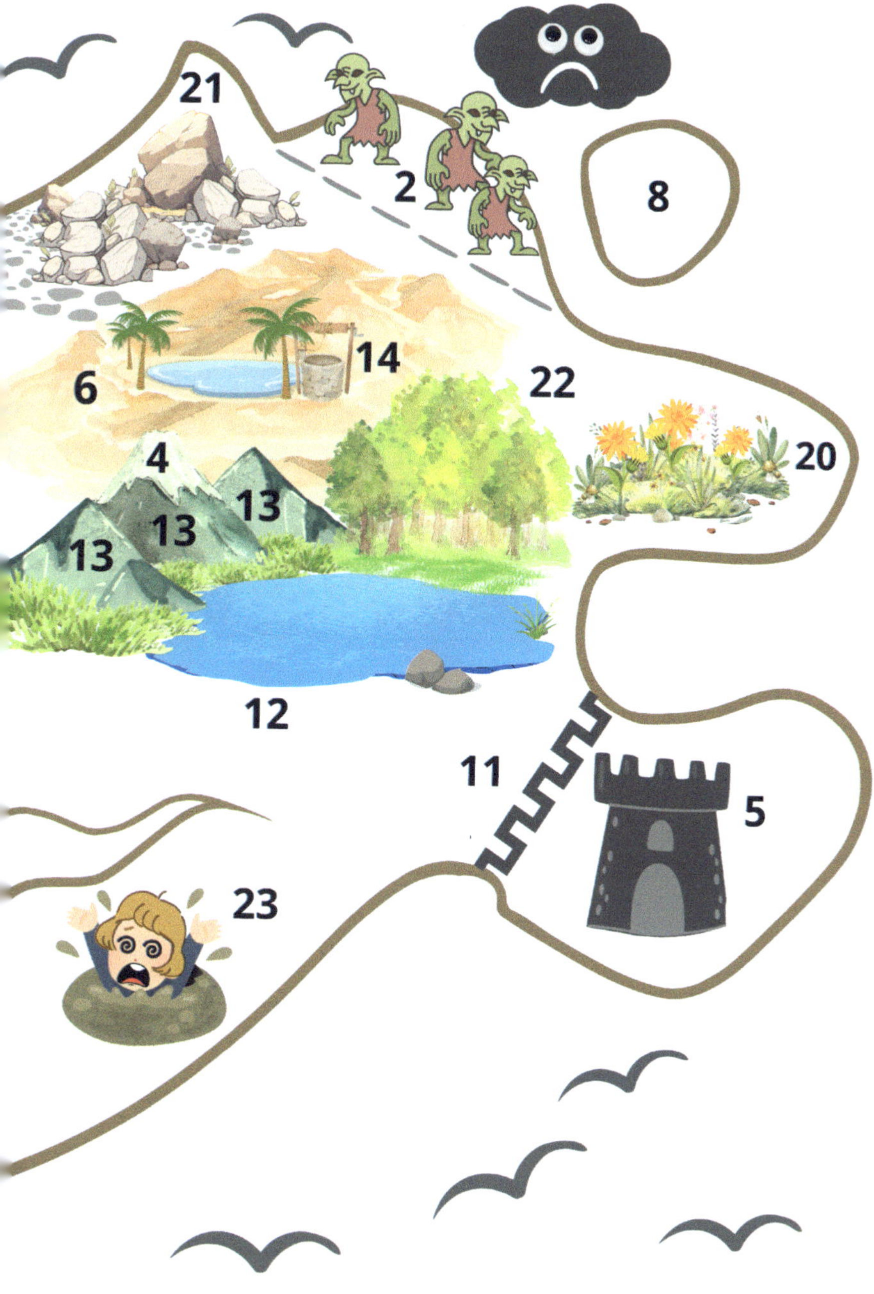
21
2
8
14
6
22
4
20
13
13
13
12
11
5
23

THE TREASURE MAP BRIEF LOCATION KEY...

1. Adrift without a Rudder
2. Anti-Life Gremlins Land
3. Bloody Burnout
4. Clear View Mountain Top
5. Clarity Castle
6. Desert
7. Doing Great Peninsula
8. Doldrums
9. Every-which-way-signpost
10. Fear Central
11. Great Wall of Self-Sabotage
12. Lake Calm
13. Mountains
14. Oasis
15. Rapids
16. River
17. Riverside Riviera
18. Steep Cliffs
19. Stuck Bog
20. Wild Flower Meadow
21. Wilderness
22. Woods
23. WTF Quick Sand

The fact that you feel discontented, frustrated, overwhelmed or lost doesn't point to you beginning your personal and spiritual growth at any specific place on the map.

You could be in the Stuck Bog, Bloody Burnout, the Desert, or fallen off the Steep Cliffs. Only you will know your existential state right now.

And if you're wondering what any of these locations feel like there's an extended key at the end of RE-DISCOVERED which describes them, together with actions you can take when you're at each one.

The Treasure Map aims to help you identify where you are as you explore who you really are, where you're going, and what you came here to do.

Knowing where you are metaphorically brings its own assurance, even if you feel crap.

"Ah, that's where I am!"

And, as actions are allocated to each location, you have a choice about how you might proceed. By the way, you might find some tips from The Treasure Map Key mentioned sporadically in other RE-DISCOVERED sections too.

In my defence, as Mae West once said, "Too much of a good thing can be wonderful!"

In identifying your location at any one time, don't logically decide it. Allow yourself to peruse the map and intuitively choose the location your eye lingers on and your index finger wants to point to as the right one right now.

Even if you don't know why, **trust your inner wisdom about that choice**. Then explore the location's description. I bet it will have meaning for you.

You can also use this map as you travel through life in general as it contains more locations than I mention in RE-DISCOVERED. Who knows how it might help you to navigate events as they occur?

If where you are doesn't appear on the map, do let me know so I can expand it. Contact me at sharon@thewildelder.com and by way of thanks I'll send you the link to my 47-Second Inner Wisdom Activator audio.

The Activator can be used when you want to connect with calmness and where you're best placed to listen to your fail-proof inner guidance. More about that later in the WHO ARE YOU? section.

Finally, **this is a map without an X marks the spot for where the treasure is buried**.[1] All will be explained at the end because what's important for the present is you're fully equipped to dive in and dive deep into Down & Dirty Spirituality right now.

ENDNOTES

1. Download your own Treasure Map in colour at www.re-discovered.life

1 DOWN & DIRTY SPIRITUALITY

WHAT SPIRITUALITY IS AND ISN'T...

What spirituality is and isn't is a great philosophical debate, but we're not going there.

There's a two-year-old wide-eyed and innocent child in me who looks at problems, contentious issues and conflicting ideologies and exclaims, "But it's so simple. All you have to do is xyz!"

When you boil things down to their essence, she's usually right. That's why we're not going there only to disappear up our proverbial with intellectual curlicues and fandangos.

Even more, if you think you're a spiritual person or the notion of spirituality feels distant and unfamiliar, welcome.

If you think you have to be religious to be spiritual or believe in a more secular reality, welcome.

If you think spirituality is all a bit woo-woo or you wholeheartedly embrace its ethereal essence, welcome.

Philosophical wrangling or what kind of person you are doesn't matter on your RE-DISCOVERED adventure. Just anticipate surprises that hopefully nudge the boundaries of your understanding.

So, let's start with what spirituality isn't...

It's nothing to do with what I call "space cadets" or the overly optimistic happy-clappy-love-and-light brigade. Flying high and only seeing yourself, others and life through rose-tinted glasses is known as "spiritual bypassing".

It's a way to avoid dealing with the down-and-dirty reality of life as a human being here on Earth.

Nor is it to do with chanting, fasting, dancing circles, being vegan, breathing through your nose in a certain way, or having to join a particular organisation to be it.

So, we won't be doing any of that!

Spirituality has nothing to do with organised religion either. It has nothing to do with the sanctity of holy water, the enchantment of specific rituals, observing certain dietary requirements, or reading particular scripts.

So, what is spirituality?

There's an old Zen saying that you can't describe the taste of sugar. The closest we can come to a definition of sugar is the word "sweet".

But what does sweet mean?

And does it convey the sensory essence of the taste of sugar?

No...

You have to put some sugar in your mouth and let your taste buds experience it to know how it tastes.

It's the same with spirituality. To truly understand it you must experience it first-hand, fully engaging your senses and emotions. Otherwise, it's nothing more than an intellectual concept.

So, how can you experience spirituality?

One way is through mystical events, voices, and visions, where you're given a message or mission to carry out. Like Joan of Arc who believed God was calling her to free her country from the English and to help the Dauphin, Charles, gain the French throne.

Luckily, I haven't had a spiritual experience that ended with me being burnt at the stake as Joan was. Instead, I've had mystical experiences that usually crept up on me unawares.

There was a time when I was unhappily married and clinically depressed. Writing that phrase made me think of being like a sausage in a too-tight skin. Ready to explode at any moment in my misery.

On a particular summer's day, I woke very early and went down to the kitchen for water. As I swung open the internal kitchen door, my breath caught in my throat.

The sun's rays were streaming fiercely and majestically straight at me through the south-facing glass back door. It felt as though I was being held by the transformative light of the Divine, like a character in some epic biblical movie.

I dropped to my knees in awe, and, as I did, I heard a deep, calm voice in my head say firmly, "I've been fighting for you!"

Huge sobs of relief wracked my body, and, in the moment, as I fell to my knees, I realised I'd been unconsciously killing myself off through starvation as you do when clinically depressed with no appetite.

That experience was a massive turning point.

Although occasionally gagging, I forced myself to eat something. My recovery and re-discovery of myself had begun!

Where did that voice come from?

Some would say God in whatever form they believed in. Some would say it was the protective voice of my guardian angel and some would say it was my constant spirit guide.

That resonant voice, for me, was and is the voice of my Wild Soul. More of that later.

Not everyone has mystical experiences of the revelation kind. But it's likely you've had a lived experience of spirituality and not known it.

Let your memory roll back to being in a beautiful place in nature. Perhaps tears prick your eyes. Perhaps you draw in a breath and feel deeply touched and even experience a sense of oneness with all that is.

A magnificent sunrise or sunset can do that for you too.

Or maybe you remember holding a newborn or young baby in your arms, mesmerised as its tiny fingers automatically curl around your one big finger and wonderment floods through you.

Or maybe there's a memory of gazing into your beloved's eyes, losing yourself in the swirl of ecstatic, deep union.

There's a good reason it's said that your eyes are the window to your soul. Look deeply-deeply straight into yours in a mirror for a while and notice what happens.

If you think this is all a bit much, the lived experience of spirituality has been confirmed by neuroscientific research. When people have lived spiritual experiences, specific areas of their brain consistently light up.[1]

It seems we humans are hardwired for spirituality whether we consciously engage with it or not.

All the above examples and more you'll read later illustrate that "what spirituality is" is simple. No faffing about. No complicated formula. No intermediary.

Spirituality is the secret sauce which makes all the difference to who you are and how you perceive yourself, others, and life, where you're going, what you do and how you do it.

Spirituality is also a relationship with the Divine.

As you develop, it's a relationship that enables you to feel safe whatever's happening in your life, to have a sense of belonging with something bigger than yourself, and to know **who you are and what you do matters**.

Indeed, it's a relationship that involves far more than lived spiritual experiences, as you'll discover.

> What does spirituality mean for you?
>
> If you've had a revelation like mine in the kitchen (and not everybody has), what was your realisation?
>
> Which spiritual lived experiences in your life stick out for you?
>
> Where are you now on the Treasure Map?

ENDNOTES

1. Miller L., *The Awakened Brain – The Psychology of Spirituality*, 2021, Penguin Random House UK

WHAT'S DOWN & DIRTY SPIRITUALITY?

If spirituality is a one-on-one relationship with the Divine involving lived spiritual experiences, what on earth is Down & Dirty Spirituality and how can it help you rediscover yourself?

Well, here's the thing…

Spend too much time at the top of a mountain and you develop altitude sickness due to the lack of oxygen.

The purpose of mountain climbing is to reach the summit, enjoy the experience, and then head back down to earth and everyday life.

As is the purpose of spirituality.

It's not all about transcendence, "going up", and one-way messages from the above. It's also coming down to earth and having a two-way relationship and communication.

Take Joan, for example. What did she do after her mystical experience, the message from the Divine? She cut her hair short, bound her breasts tightly, and passed herself off as a male soldier to fight in the war.

That was sensible, in that no way could she fulfil the mission as a young French peasant girl, and it was also a message to the Divine.

Over and out.

I've got this!

In a nutshell, **Down & Dirty Spirituality is reaching the heights, transcending your normal experience, and bringing any learning or transformation down to earth by expressing it in everyday life.**

And you do that through your personality with two feet firmly on the ground. Indeed, the process of earthly expression is known in the trade as "grounding!"

It's making real the philosophical concepts of "as in heaven, here on earth" and "as above so below".

Ultimately, you create your own heaven or hell right here on Earth.

I look back on my life as a child right up to my early thirties when I was living unconsciously. A bundle of beliefs, attitudes, and behaviours that had formed unconsciously through what had happened to me; the creature I was conditioned to be rather than the being I was designed to be.

I was like a robot working on automatic. What I call "living dead". And the hell I was unconsciously creating was predicated on my earlier life, memories of which are mostly unhappy.

My parents were children themselves who never should have had children. Both were abusive in their way through ignorance, operating unconsciously themselves as a result of what had happened to them.

They were blindly repeating inter-generational patterns of behaviour.

While I can remember snippets of happy times, like beside the seaside, mostly I remember my parents bickering or arguing ferociously, creating their version of hell. My mother was asleep a lot of the time as a result of heavy-duty drugs used in the 1950s to "cure" depression.

So, reading books and being at school saved me; both nourishing escapes in different ways.

I must have been the only child in the school who hated school holidays and couldn't wait for school to start again!

Well, perhaps not. I wouldn't have recognised others like me way back then.

BUT...

Being able to create your own heaven or hell here on Earth means that however shit you feel right now there's always hope.

You might be in the Doldrums, on the edge of Steep Cliffs or in Bloody Burnout. Wherever you are on the Treasure

Map, Down & Dirty Spirituality's therapeutic work will help you.

How?

Firstly, there's no analysis or psychobabble.

For example, a mentee of mine was told by her therapist she was suffering "disenfranchised grief".

What the ... is that?

Her therapist could have said something more useful like, "I'm wondering whether you feel other people don't recognise your loss or allude to you not grieving in the right way?"

You're having a difficult enough time as it is. Who needs jargon that usually only the therapist understands?

Secondly, there are no contorted psychological or spiritual theories in Down & Dirty Spirituality. SIMPLICITY is economical and effective.

As Albert Einstein said, "If you can't explain it to a six-year-old, you don't understand it yourself."

All techniques used in Down & Dirty Spirituality collaborate with the way you're wired up.

Take the technique of Evocative Words. OK, I'll give you that sounds a bit like jargon, but it does say what it does on the tin.

Say you need more fun in your life. Write "fun" on a load of Post-its. Plaster them around your home and wherever you'll be. From your dashboard to your undies drawer to your work diary and so on.

From the Post-it, you absorb the word "fun" visually which echoes in your head auditorily until you don't even notice you're reading it anymore.

In effect, it becomes a mantra to which the brain responds with, "Oh, you want some more fun in your life? I'll work on it!"

Not long after you'll notice you are having more fun. You'll have evoked the quality of fun into your life for real.

Yes, I did look for neuroscientific proof for the efficacy of the technique, but, hey, it was so complex and inconclusive that I gave up! As they say on some herbal supplements, what I've said about the effectiveness of the Evocative Words technique is "based on traditional use only".

But, take it from me, it works!

Thirdly, in Down & Dirty Spirituality, there's no trawling through your history looking for trouble.

No urging you to find and re-experience trauma. No getting you to access pain to relive it in the here and now. Of course, something historic can pop up and when it does, we work with it in the present to improve your life now and your future.

You are in charge of the process and if you need to stop at any time you just stop.

If we were working together, I would never encourage you to do anything that didn't feel right. I might well ask what happened to make you stop doing something as it's usually a valuable piece of your process which we might explore further, but that's all.

Lastly, Down & Dirty Spirituality is all about you being your own expert even if you don't know that or think you can't be.

For a start, you hold shedloads of information you're unaware of. Some of it's great and some of it's not so great, but ALL information about you, conscious or unconscious, is fuel for your growth and highest good.

Plus, with Down & Dirty Spirituality, you only work with what's immediately at "the top of the pile", the thing that feels most important to explore in the moment.

Because, when you resolve the thing at the top of the pile, there's a positive trickle-down effect on issues beneath it. Needless to say, this is economical for your time, effort, and finances if you're paying for therapy.

And how do you do all that?

Many therapeutic ways of using Down & Dirty Spirituality are sprinkled throughout RE-DISCOVERED, including the power and mystery of your magnificent imagination.

Which do you prefer, reaching the heights or having two feet firmly on the ground, and why?

How could you apply Down & Dirty Spirituality to your life?

What could change for the better if you did, and why?

Where are you now on the Treasure Map?

IMAGINATION AND A RESOURCE FOR YOUR ADVENTURE

I was thirteen and feeling lost possibly for the first time. I can remember feeling lonely, not fitting in with how the girls at my youth club behaved, and wanting to be a boy.

Not just wanting but desperately longing to be a boy!

I hung around with them at the youth club. I cultivated a boyish swagger and swore as only young teenage boys do. They humoured me for a while, possibly amused by my oddity. However, it wasn't long before they told me in no uncertain terms where to go.

I was bereft, thrown back into my lost discontent and the darkness I now recognise as depression.

What motivated my passionate desire to be a boy?

It was only in later life when in therapy that I realised the cause. I'd seen being powerful and active in the world as the prerogative of the males in the immediate family in which I was raised.

That wasn't unusual with the gender zeitgeist of the 1950s and '60s whatever they tell you about swinging Britain!

However, that was even more so in my family. My grandfather and uncle were market traders and always came home with great animated stories, lighting up the general dreariness.

Their behaviour and reality were set against the women's in stark relief.

My mother and grandmother didn't work outside the home, and didn't do much of anything else either, including housework.

They were passive and generally depressed. Although I remember my mother creating exquisite embroidery, this activity didn't last long.

Nothing did!

No wonder I unconsciously rejected a woman's lot as my future. No wonder I made an unconscious decision that I wanted to be a boy.

It wasn't until my forties, working with my unconscious as a very masculine identified woman, that I began a journey of reclaiming the feminine aspects of myself I had previously shut down.

Including the delicious Divine Feminine!

If you're able to access unconscious drivers, you can always mend what you can mend and learn to manage the rest. In this way, you can change your behaviour and align yourself more with who you were designed to be rather than who you were conditioned to be.

So, how on earth do you work with your unconscious?

Socrates (490–399 BC) was one of the earliest to recognise that there is more to us than meets the eye.[1]

Fast forward to Sigmund Freud (1856–1939) who publicised the idea that your behaviour is driven by your "unconscious", which is formed by childhood events and significant experiences in your life. Most, if not all, of which you don't remember.

Deliciously for our purposes, he found a relatively easy way to work with the unconscious through analysing dreams. As he said, "The interpretation of dreams is the royal road to a knowledge of the unconscious activities of the mind."[2]

Now, I'm not going to ask you to disappear up the Mountains where the air is rarified, there are no distractions, and you can focus 1000% on interpreting your dreams.

There's an even easier way to access your unconscious.

And that is through daydreaming!

As I don't know a woman who hasn't at some time daydreamed about something or someone she's desired, this is very doable for you.

And when you daydream, you do so through your imagination which creates mental images or concepts of what isn't present to your senses in reality.

I rest my case!

Through your imagination, you can access vital unconscious information for your adventure from feeling discontented, lost, or adrift to rediscovering who you really are, where you're going, and what you came here to do.

If you think you don't dream or that imagination isn't one of your strengths, no problem!

Some people imagine in technicolour images like they're seeing a movie. I usually don't "see" anything, but I get a "sense" of what's going on in my imagination, often followed by "hearing" something like a word or a snatch of a song.

However you imagine (even if you think you don't) is the right way to imagine for you. All of which is great because you'll be using imagination a fair bit in your re-discovery adventure!

The glorious thing about imagination is that, while it sometimes gives you understandable information, it uses whatever it can to communicate information.

It will use metaphors, symbols, song tunes, physical sensations, place names, advertising boards, overheard conversations, anything, but anything, from this universe or outside it.

So, when using your imagination, take whatever you get even if it seems nonsensical or bizarre.

Censor nothing however ridiculous it might seem to you and your logical mind.

Everything you imagine is a clue to something. And the clues often need to accumulate for you to get that "Ah, now I know what it means" moment.

Why isn't the process easier? Why don't you just receive the information you need to grow in a straightforward way?

Who knows, except maybe the Divine!

That's why I often tell my clients, if there's somewhere to go after I'm physically dead, I'm going to have a word with the management. Surely "they" could have made the process less complicated...

ENOUGH!

It's time to receive a resource through a guided daydream that can support you on your RE-DISCOVERED adventure.[3]

Sit comfortably upright with your feet on the floor. Close your eyes and take three deep breaths in and out, releasing any tension in your body.

Focus deep down into your belly, tilting your chin downward just a little and take three more deep breaths.

Now, imagine you're in a beautiful safe meadow on a warm summer's day, a cool breeze gently caressing your skin.

Explore your beautiful safe meadow with all of your senses.

What can you see?

What can you hear?

What can you smell?

What are the textures under your fingers?

And how do you feel?

Now notice a wizened old tree nearby. Notice its branches are full of life, resplendent with the green of its leaves.

As you move towards it, your eyes are drawn to a hole in its trunk that seems to be calling you.

As you move closer, you know instinctively that the resource you need for your RE-DISCOVERED adventure awaits you in the tree trunk through that hole.

And you know whatever the resource is, however bizarre or nonsensical it could appear, however big or small it is, whether you understand what it is or not, this is the right resource for you.

So, reach into the hole and take your resource in whatever image, shape, or form it appears to you.

Thank the tree and sit somewhere in your beautiful safe meadow where you can explore your resource.

Take time to familiarise yourself with it.

Then, taking your resource with you, allow your experience of the meadow to fade.

Turn your attention slowly outward, twiddle your fingers and toes, or stretch if need be, and, when you're ready, gently open your eyes, and come back into the room.

If you feel a bit light-headed or not quite back in your body, rub your limbs fiercely and your chest, thorax, and belly. Jump up and down ten times until you feel back in your body and the room.

BTW if you got nothing, be chill about it. Nothing is something in its own way.

In this case, just sit with your nothing and sense its qualities, textures, and colours if it had them. Explore all of its qualities and see what emerges.

Congratulations!

You've just connected with your inner wisdom and spiritual intelligence through your imagination. You've found your resource. If you don't consciously understand what it is or its meaning, you will in the hours or days to come.

Create a drawing of your resource, or write what it is, on a card that you can display as a reminder. That will support and motivate you in your adventure as you move forward.

With a taste of what spirituality is, my Down & Dirty version, and having limbered up your imagination, you're now well equipped to explore who you really are right now.

> In what way or ways do you imagine?
>
> What's your resource and how can it support you?
>
> If you got nothing, return to it momentarily and explore its qualities and what, if anything, emerged from it.
>
> Where are you now on the Treasure Map?

ENDNOTES

1. Dijksterhuis A., The Unconscious, Libre Texts, Social Sciences, https://socialsci.libretexts.org/Bookshelves/Psychology/Introductory_Psychology/Psychology_(Noba)/Chapter_7%3A_Cognition_and_Language/7.2%3A_The_Unconscious (Accessed 1 February 2024)
2. The Interpretation of Dreams, Freud Museum London, https://www.freud.org.uk/education/resources/the-interpretation-of-dreams/ (Accessed 1 February 2024)
3. Access an unabridged audio version of the Your RE-DISCOVERED Adventure Resource at www.re-discovered.life

2 WHO ARE YOU?

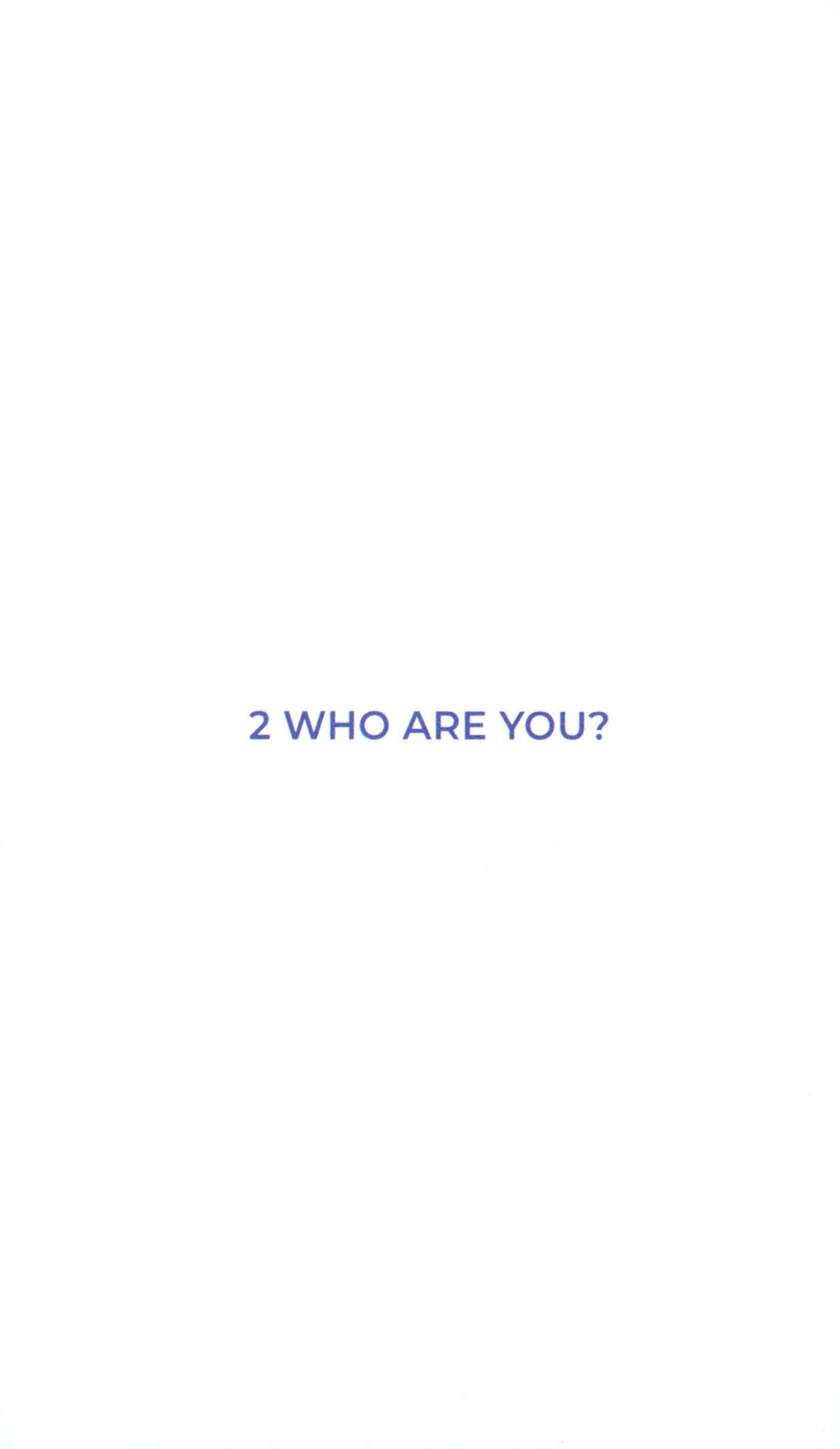

YOUR PERSONALITY

I'd decided that Earth was a penal colony by the time I turned fourteen. I was sure I'd done something very wrong somewhere else in the universe to have come to the living hell I was experiencing!

Existing in my grandparents' home with its depressed energy, my mother was absent even when she was there, and I had no connection with my younger sister at all. I felt unheld, unloved, and alone.

Always an outsider looking in.

To cap it all, the local grammar school I attended offered lacklustre instruction for a girl who could fly with unicorns.

I rebelled.

I truanted.

I wasn't just discontented.

I was lost and Adrift Without a Rudder, fearful this was how life would always be...

Feeling discontented, lost, or adrift, or any of their associated feelings, can be overwhelming. It seems as though every single cell in your body has been hijacked and shackled.

You can end up thinking WHO YOU ARE is lost, adrift, overwhelmed, or whatever feeling demands to be felt at any particular moment.

And, if you're doing an "I'm fine!" cover-up, it leaves you feeling even more disconnected and isolated.

You could experience yourself in the middle of the Wilderness or the Desert, going over the Rapids, or even on the Great Wall of Self-sabotage.

It doesn't matter where you are.

The overriding thought is, "How the hell can I get out of this?"

Escape seems impossible!

However, the good news is who you are is never how you're feeling in the moment, although it might seem like it.

You'll also confuse who you are with your personality which is a bundle of thoughts, feelings, beliefs, attitudes, and behaviour. All necessary to function in the material world in which we live. But even then…

Your personality is not just one ongoing entity as I thought it was when I was fourteen.

For example, the way you relate to and behave with a loved one, a shop assistant, and a work colleague will differ enormously. Unless, of course, they comprise a highly unlikely combo!

Instead, you're made up of many different parts, or sub-personalities, each with a life of its own.

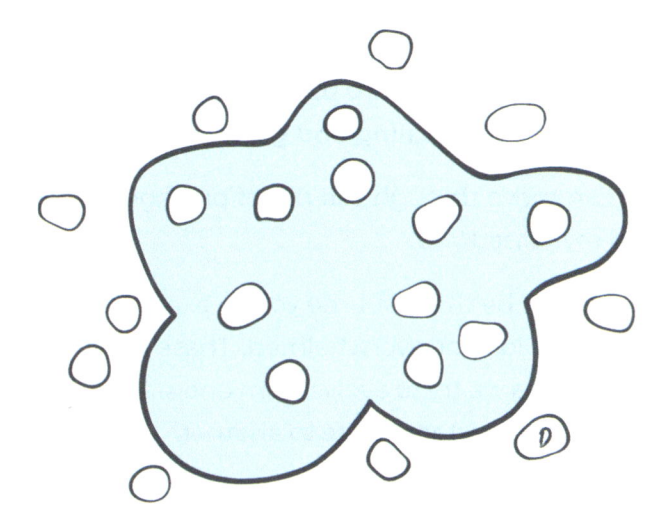

The "amoeba" looking graphic represents **the boundary of your consciousness within which lies your "core" personality.** These are the parts of you you know about and like. It also contains parts of you you don't like and prefer to keep hidden.

For example, some of the parts of me that I like are the teacher, the mother, the old crone and, deliciously, as I write RE-DISCOVERED, I'm enjoying the writer. Some of the parts of me I don't like are the whiner, the self-sabotager, and the nagger.

The blobs outside of the boundary represent parts of your personality about which you're unconscious. You have no idea they exist. And it's usually one of those parts that feels discontented, lost or adrift, or whatever allied feeling you major in at any particular moment.

The reason for it being uppermost is it's **the feeling of a part of you trying very hard to get your attention so you work with it for its healing and growth**.

So you can move through the rite of passage it's offering you to a revitalised you.

This might not be the first time you've experienced being discontented, lost, or overwhelmed. These feeling states are common as we try to evolve from one state of being to another, from one stage of life to another.

It's like you're wearing old worn-out clothes that are disintegrating before your very eyes, but your new ones haven't yet been sewn together. And you have no idea what they'll look like!

I remember that happening to me in my thirties. Having been uber-identified with masculine parts of me, it felt as if tectonic plates were shifting when feminine aspects of me cried out for attention.

To say I felt uncomfortable is an under-statement!

I felt like I could rip my chest open with my bare hands and yell like a demented Tarzaness. Every masculine sinew in me strained against welcoming in a softer, more sensitive, and more flowing energy.

I feared being as vulnerable as a child if I dared to let down my masculine guard.

Even more, I feared losing control as if I would end up running down the High Road waving my knickers in the air while yelling in tongues!

Also, when you're in transition facing the unknown, **it's not unusual for scared or even terrified parts of you to come to the fore, screaming for attention.**

Believe me, if you want to give yourself the heebie-jeebies, challenge yourself to write a book. Here's one of my social media posts from January 2024 while writing RE-DISCOVERED…

> "I'm struggling with this every freakin' day right now…
>
> It's not as if I don't know what's behind it…
>
> The sexually abused little girl who was told to keep the secret… or else!
>
> The sexually, mentally and emotionally abused little girl who had nightmares about WTF the warning "or else" could mean.
>
> The bright, talented girl who would say, write and create "unexpected" things!
>
> I eventually learned not to put my head above the parapet "What an actress you are!" "Ooo-er look at you!"

Ridiculed and humiliated, I unconsciously hid her creativity in fear of its destruction.

The serious deep girl with a Wild Soul endangered by her mother's jealousy, the fallout of World War III between her parents and the manipulations of a toxic grandmother.

So, I hid her light too.

I've been chipping away at fears about being visible for a long while with some success...

BUT...

Now at 75, as I challenge myself to write my legacy book, initiate a sacred spiritual growth group for women AND be seen widely as the magnificent and powerfully effective spiritual psychotherapist coach that I am...

THESE AND ALL MY OTHER VISIBILITY FEARS HAVE COALESCED!

My forty years' professional expertise, knowledge, and wisdom tell me those fears are in their death throes... A final cumulative assault to keep me silent and invisible.

My Wild Soul and I and the sacred work I offer are too precious to be silenced any more!

This post is my public and sacred declaration that, despite the grinding dread in the pit of my stomach

> and the nausea rising in my throat, **I WILL NOT FREA-KIN' SUCCUMB ANY MORE!**
>
> I invoke the awesome and healing energy of love.
>
> I forgive myself for feeling fear – I CHOOSE LOVE INSTEAD!
>
> SO IT IS, so it is, and so it is…"

Different parts of me that carried fears about visibility, putting my head above the parapet, had joined forces to stop me from writing RE-DISCOVERED.

There's no doubt I was in Fear Central, and I stopped writing for several weeks until I got wise to what was going on. By the end of my post, you'll notice the mantra, "I forgive myself for feeling fear and I choose love instead."

The good news is Love and fear cannot co-exist, and so Love is the perfect antidote to fear.

Some women imagine Love's powerful and healing energy like seeing moonbeams emanating from a night's sky. Some women imagine it as Tinkerbell's fairy dust. Whatever way you imagine the energy of Love to look and be, use that in this experiment.[1]

Take a few deep breaths. Gently close your eyes and see or sense the part of you that's felt fearful in the past or feels fearful right now.

Take whatever you get however bizarre.

If you get nothing, that's OK. Proceed as if you have.

Now, imagine a rainfall showerhead above your fearful part very gently showering it with the magnificent and healing energy of Love.

See or sense Love cascading down from the top of your fearful part until it's entirely cocooned in Love's healing energy.

Gently, gently...

Feel yourself soften and relax, soften and relax, soften and relax...

Then, thanking the healing energy of Love, allow what you're seeing or sensing to fade, turn your attention outward again, gently open your eyes, and come back into the room.

You've just changed how you felt from fear to feeling something preferable. How on earth did you do that?

Well, imagine your personality made of many different parts is an orchestra limbering up before a performance.

If you've ever experienced that, you'll know each instrument makes whatever sounds it likes, and the net result is a cacophony of chaotic sound.

In the same way, different parts of you make their own sounds willy-nilly, including the part of you that feels discontented, lost, or overwhelmed.

All clamouring to be heard over the others.

We'll explore how you can stop the noise and orchestrate your personality parts to play beautifully in tune in the next section, "You are more than your personality."

> Draw your own "core personality" diagram and name those parts you know about, those you like and those you don't.
>
> When you showered your fearful part with the healing energy of Love, what happened?
>
> If you had to guess, what parts of you could be outside your core personality?
>
> Where are you now on the Treasure Map?

ENDNOTES

1. Access the audio for The Love and Fear Experiment at www.re-discovered.life

YOU ARE MORE THAN YOUR PERSONALITY

It was early morning when I woke agitated and couldn't get back to sleep during a bout of depression. I got up for some reason and when I returned I lay down, using a breathing sequence which causes your nervous system to calm down.[1]

I focused on my breathing, counting each inhalation, exhalation, and pause and then...

Something incredible happened!

I heard the deep slow breathing pattern you hear when you lie next to someone fast asleep. Only it wasn't someone else. It was my breathing.

It was me hearing me sleeping.

It was so weird and anyone could be forgiven for feeling scared, like WTF is going on? But I wasn't scared. There was a stillness about me, and, **in that moment, I realised there was far more to me than I thought.**

And I was right!

You need your body, feelings, mind, and personality to navigate our world of form and matter. They're like the components of an awesome spacesuit in which you can live safely, depending on how well each component operates.

However, my experience that morning made me realise that **I am so much more than my body, more than my feelings, more than my mind, and more than my personality.**

So are you!

What you are in essence is pure consciousness, just like the pure consciousness that was observing me asleep that morning.

That might sound a bit space cadet-like if you're a cynic, so here's how my Down & Dirty Spirituality sees it...

At essence, you have a Wild Soul.

This is your Spark of the Divine within and also your connection to the Divine without, Universe, God, Goddess, The Way, Brahman, whatever your name for whatever you perceive as a bigger, greater force for good in our solar system and beyond.

Your Wild Soul carries your original design.

Think of that as your assigned Divine homework. A unique template of your potential to develop who you are, where you're going, and what you came here to be and do.

Writing that reminded me of "This Be The Verse," a cynical poem by Philip Larkin that starts, "They fuck you up, your Mum and Dad." [2]

But, hey, it's not just them.

From birth, you're socialised and conditioned to be whatever's "acceptable" in the tribe, wider culture, and country in which you were born.

Potential?

What's potential?

There's an old rabbinical story that **when the Divine was creating humans she was in a quandary about where to put our Wild Soul.**

One angel said, "Put it at the top of the highest mountain. They'll never think of finding it there!"

Another angel said, "Put it at the bottom of the deepest ocean. They'll never think of finding it there."

And yet another angel said, "Naaa (or similar!) eventually they'll go to the top of the highest mountain and the bottom of the deepest ocean. Put their Wild Soul inside of them. They'll never think of looking for it there!"

And, until we get shown or stumble upon it by chance, as I did, the angel was absolutely right!

Plus, because your Wild Soul carries your original design, it instinctively knows what's right for you and not right for you, and communicates this through the voice of its inner wisdom.

On the morning of my wedding 90,000 years ago, I felt sick, sick, sick to my stomach, and then I heard a huge loud NOOOOOO inside my head.

Did I listen?

I did not.

I put the whole thing down to pre-wedding nerves and forged ahead into nineteen years of all that not being with the right person for me entailed.

Did I learn a lot and grow because of that marriage?

Sure, I did.

We can learn and grow through anything that occurs in our lives.

However, with hindsight, I realised that, on that fateful morning, I was receiving heavy-duty advice from my Wild Soul's inner wisdom not to go ahead with the wedding.

Now, if you think of your Wild Soul as a blazing summer sun, you'll know you can't look directly at it without damaging your eyes.

So, very cleverly **you have a Spark of your Wild Soul at the level of your personality for everyday use.**

It observes what's happening in your life non-judgementally, and can spur you into action when needed.

In the next graphic you'll see something's changed.

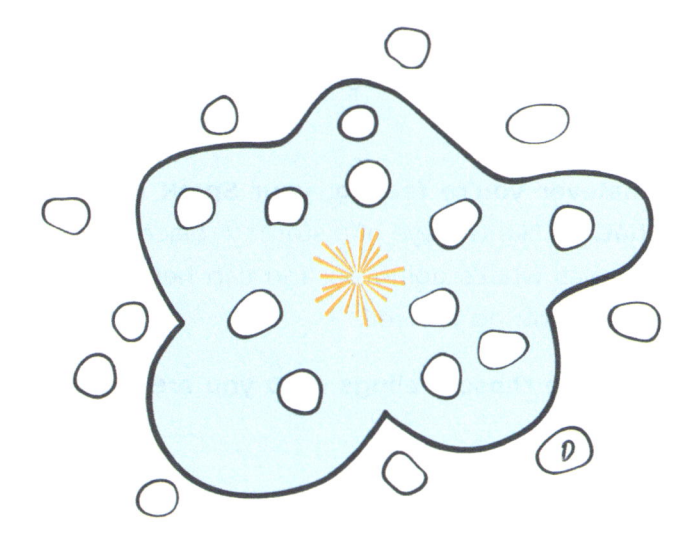

Remember that unruly orchestra from the core personality diagram?

Your "Spark" is that orchestra's conductor.

Instead of seeing it in the middle of your personality, imagine looking down at your Spark in the diagram from above so you can appreciate that it's separate and different from your personality in its nature.

When it exerts its influence, it enables your personality parts to collaborate and make sweet sweet music.

Well, some of the time!

Your Spark can also do more if you collaborate with it.

For example, take the "discontented" part of your personality about which you've previously been unconscious. It's marked with a D in the diagram.

That part could be caught up or overwhelmed with feeling Adrift Without a Rudder or be in Fear Central or WTF Quick Sand.

But, whatever you're feeling, your Spark is separate from that. It's like the eye of a storm. A place of stillness that observes what's going on and can help you make choices like centring yourself.

Yes, you have those feelings AND you are more than your feelings.

Your Wild Soul's inner wisdom knows your discontented part is playing up because it needs your attention for its healing and growth. And by centring in your Spark you can begin that process.

How?

Through a process of non-judgemental observation of your discontented part and taking specific action to build a reparative relationship with it.

Take a minute to imagine your discontented part and how it would look if you could see or sense it.

Remember this is imaginary work so accept whatever you get however bizarre it might seem.

Now, start building a relationship with it by exploring how that part of you presents to your senses.

How does it look and feel to your touch?

How would it sound if it spoke?

How would it smell and even taste?

What's its temperature, hot, normal, or cold?

I know! Don't worry if you don't get answers for some of the above. Just trust your process that's working whether you're aware of it or not.

Think of it like dating and getting to know that part of you so well that, in time, you'll finish its sentences and predict its reactions and responses.

When you know it this well, you'll have a choice as to whether you do or say what you've always done or do or say something different and more productive.

As Einstein once intimated, if you keep on doing what you've always done and expect something different to happen, you're whistling in the wind!

A beneficial change in what you do or say is the only way forward if you desire healing and growth.

The awesome thing is that if you ask any personality part what it needs to heal and grow, it will usually tell you.

By the way, what it needs is never a "thing" or a "want" like "three bars of chocolate." If you get an answer like that, dig deeper.

Because your part's need will always be a spiritual quality of being like Love, Safety, Understanding, or Compassion.[3]

And please don't assume you know how your part needs to experience that spiritual quality.

Ask it the question!

For example, with the quality of Love, it could be hugs, or adult you just being there, or being wrapped in a big duvet or, or, or... absolutely anything.

The discontented part of you froze way back in your history because it wasn't given and nourished with that particular spiritual quality. So it stayed frozen until you could give it what it needed.

It waited for a time when "adult you" could reparent it, melt it back to warmth and good health, and bring it home into your core personality.

And remember, while the Spark of your Wild Soul orchestrates this sacred process from within, you can also be held and supported by the Divine without too!

> Journal about a personality part you came across while reading this section.
>
> What does knowing you're more than you thought you were mean for you?
>
> How would your life change if you could use your Spark to choose what you say and do?
>
> Where are you now on the Treasure Map?

ENDNOTES

1. Access the breathing sequence audio at www.re-discovered.life
2. Larkin P., *Collected Poems*, 2003, Faber & Faber
3. Access What Are Your Spiritual Qualities? at www.re-discovered.life

YOUR CONNECTION WITH THE DIVINE

Over forty years ago I was falling apart. I had wanted to be a clinical psychologist for years. But when I became disillusioned by the kind of psychology taught in my degree programme, that was the last thing I wanted to be.

I was left not knowing who I was, where I was going, and definitely not what I'd come here to do!

Believe it or believe it not, psychotherapy was then in its infancy in the UK. So, I had to travel all the way from outer East London to the frontiers of North London to have therapy with someone recommended to me.

It was a schlep!

A whole day out of my week, given travelling time there and back and the ninety-minute appointment.

My therapist hired a therapy room in a house that was a long walk from the tube station. The road the house sat in had so many trees it was avenue-like and one summer's day…

One amazing summer's day, I turned onto that road and OMG!

That avenue of trees popped with a depth of colour and texture I had never seen before.

The greens were emerald jewels dazzling in the sunshine.

The tree barks varied in colour and I saw them like cinnamon sticks and sleek brown otter skins gleaming in the weft and the warp of that road.

It was like I was tripping on some enhancing drug.

However, my therapist explained that **I'd had a "peak experience", a heightened sense of wonder, awe, or ecstasy in the normal every day.**[1]

Two years later, with the same therapist, I was going through some crap and said to him, "I wish I could have one of those peak experiences again!"

He looked at me a bit sideways and assured me that I still had them, but I'd just got used to experiencing them.

They'd become the new normal.

So, when I walked back to the station I looked consciously at that avenue of trees, and he was right. When I 100% mindfully focused on them by being very present, it was fireworks time again!

I re-experienced awe and wonder, and, in those moments, I felt deeply connected and belonging to a wondrous and benevolent energy which I call the Divine.

I've no doubt you've had at least one peak experience in your life; a deep connection in nature, holding a newborn, looking into the eyes of your beloved.

I once even had a peak experience looking at the most curvy, sexy vase I'd ever seen.

Peak experiences can be triggered by anything and everything.

They are the absolute opposite of how you experience things feeling disconnected or lost. These feelings can deepen into loss of control, chaos or even "the dark night of the soul".[2]

The dark night of the soul is a spiritual depression which you might experience in the Wilderness or the Desert where bleakness and disconnection with yourself, others, and the Divine can eat away at you.

Now, I'm not suggesting you pop a peak experience as an antidote.

It wouldn't work anyway. To ask you to go from feeling deeply disconnected to awe and wonder would be like asking you to ascend the Himalayas in one leap!

However, **you can remember your peak experience, and hold it like a candle flame, a light reminding you that who you are is so much more than this dark night of the soul.**

As with all things, this too shall pass.

Indeed, your peak experience can be an aide memoire that the wheel of life is always turning and nothing is permanent unless you choose to make it so.

And what if feeling discontented or lost was a rite of passage to rediscover more of who you were designed to be? The details of which have been suppressed or repressed because of who you were conditioned to be?

Hold that thought...

Remember the Spark of your Wild Soul that can orchestrate your busy personality? Here it is in the next diagram showing its connection to your Wild Soul.

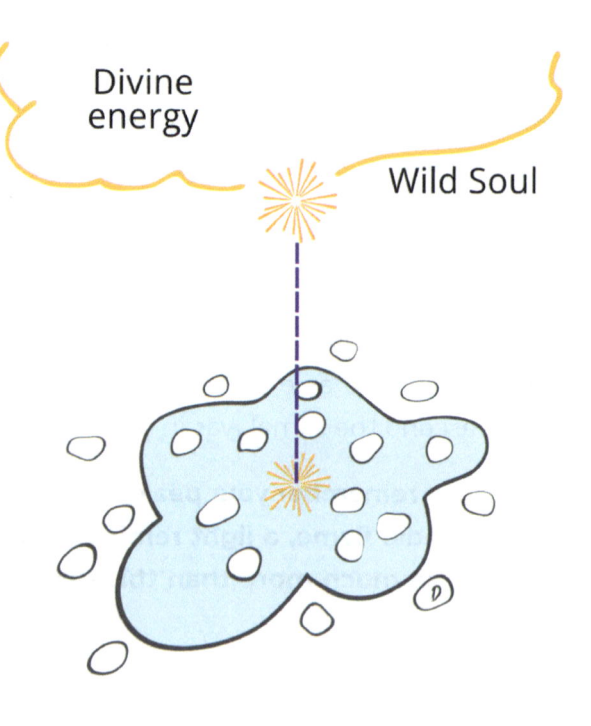

And your Wild Soul is also a connection to that wondrous and benevolent Divine energy *outside* of you!

That means there's a direct connection between you and the Divine!

Think of it this way…

In the early days of the telephone, if you wanted to speak with someone in another country, your call had to go through numerous telephone exchanges and lines.

And the connection could be easily lost if one bit of the call journey wasn't synced exactly right.

However, today, you can have a direct line from your mobile to call anyone around the world without fearing disconnection.

Similarly, you can have a direct line from your Spark through your Wild Soul to the Divine within and without *and* back again in a two-way connection!

So, what if your personality feeling discontented is your Wild Soul's evolutionary push to grow closer to the Divine so you can manifest some of your sacred potential?

What if you're not only connected to the Divine, but you're a whole freakin' manifestation of the Divine herself?

If your mind just blew up at that idea, it's because it likes to control things. Ever since Descartes's proposition, "I think, therefore I am,"[3] the status of our logical mind got elevated until it perceived itself as king over our feelings and senses.

It is, of course, deluded!

While the logical mind is excellent at rationality, analysis, and making lists, it can only go so far.

When it comes to questions of who you are, where you're going, and what you came here to do, **you need to riff along the line of your connection with the Divine for answers that speak to the magnificence and sacredness of who you really are...**

> What peak experiences have you had?
>
> How would you describe your relationship with the Divine?
>
> What would perceiving yourself as a manifestation of the Divine herself do for you?
>
> Where are you now on the Treasure Map?

ENDNOTES

1. Maslow A., On Peak Experience – The Mystical Experience, Health Policy Politics, YouTube https://www.youtube.com/watch?v=1Y4ubyz3fbY (Accessed 19 February 2024)
2. Regan S., Understanding the Dark Night of the Soul (+ How to Get Through it), mgbmindfulness https://www.mindbodygreen.com/articles/dark-night-of-soul (Accessed 4 May 2024)
3. Descartes R., Discourse on Method, 1637, Britannica https://www.britannica.com/topic/cogito-ergo-sum (Accessed 4 May 2024)

3 WHERE ARE YOU GOING?

A "before you read this section" note!

If you get clear answers to the questions in this whole section... great!

If you don't, please don't throw your hands up in despair and contemplate drastic measures or think it's all over.

The nature of the work is that you don't necessarily get clear answers immediately.

They can filter through later while you're having a shower, driving your car, in the middle of your exercise sequence... Just about anywhere any time!

So, keep a notebook handy at all times or record what you get on your mobile. Because when you get an insight you think you'll remember it but you rarely do.

Don't ask me why!

It's another one of those inscrutable growth realities which, when I'm physically dead, I'll have a word with the management about.

Be assured, if you get absolutely nothing in this section or any other, **by going through the process you're limbering up the mechanics of what will eventually deliver the answers you need** to rediscover your way forward.

Remember, you now have an advantage.

Having a better sense of who you are, having accessed your Wild Soul and its inner wisdom, and your personality conductor Spark with its ability for observation and action, **you're perfectly set up to make a list of your skills and where you've come from.**

WHERE HAVE YOU COME FROM?

The shock nearly had me go out of my mind when I heard, by chance, that my son's father with whom we were living was emigrating to South Africa in a few months.

In effect, he was dumping us!

My son was 18 months old and I was nearly 20. A grammar school girl dropout with no marketable skills to talk of but an immediate and desperate need to get some.

So, I enrolled at night school. Then, with four months' shorthand and typing skills under my belt, **I conned my way into being a secretary and learned how to do it on the job.**

It was enough to pay the rent and bills in a flat share. It also paid for my son's nursery, food, and clothes, but not for me to buy lunch at work.

We survived… just about!

I went on to make a career out of it, ending up as a PA, but it wasn't the job of my dreams. And, in my early 30s, I embarked on a psychology degree, **swearing I would never ever use shorthand and typing again.**

Little did I know…

Some two years later my then husband, having remortgaged our house to set him up in business, ruined said business spectacularly. Those very skills I swore never to use again helped put food in our mouths and clothes on our backs until we downsized our home to pay off debts and begin again.

So never say never!

Firstly, create a list of all your skills, past and present. Include domestic goddess or surrogate mother to siblings, CEO, athletics medal winner, ace bread maker, or pole dancer.

Include anything but ANYTHING that comes into your head as a skill, however bizarre. These prompts are part of defining and refining the rest of this section and everything is valuable.

Secondly, create a list headed "Where have I come from?"

Your answers to this could include ethnicity, sexual orientation, lifestyle, your ancestral line… ABSOLUTELY ANYTHING you get when you ask yourself again and again the question, "Where have I come from?"

If you get what seems ridiculous, take that too.

An answer I got a while back was that I came from, "The beat of a badger's wing on a sunny day!"

How preposterous is that?

Later, I understood it as part of what I call my down-and-dirty natural energies.

Journal every answer you get for each list over a few days, a week, or a fortnight. Whatever time it takes for you to sense you've downloaded everything needed.

If in doubt, just ask yourself, "Am I cooked?"

Your inner wisdom will either respond affirmatively or not. Follow its lead.

And when you are cooked, create a quiet and undisturbed time for the next piece of work using your lists.

When you're ready, take some deep breaths and call on your Wild Soul to hold and guide you. Working superfast to avoid your logical mind interfering in your choices, **intuitively cross through anything on each list you need to leave behind.**

If you catch yourself thinking something like, "It's not sensible to leave that behind," stand up, shake your body, and then get to it again as quickly as you can.

This is not about being sensible.

It's about chasing down where you're going.

When you've been through your lists crossing out, go and do something else for at least an hour before you come back to them.

Again, take some deep breaths and call on your Wild Soul to hold and guide you.

Then, working superfast again to avoid your logical mind interfering, **this time circle those things you instinctively find very attractive on each list.**

Don't censor or second guess what you're doing. Trust your inner wisdom, your eyes, and your hand to show you the most attractive items on each list.

When you've finished circling, turn a page in your journal and write just one list of everything you've circled from both lists.

Congratulations!

You've stirred up the juices of where you're going.

> Were you surprised by anything you crossed out and, if so, why?
>
> Were you surprised by anything you circled and, if so, why?
>
> In each case, what might that mean for where you're going?
>
> Where are you now on the Treasure Map?

ENDNOTES

1. Maslow A., On Peak Experience – The Mystical Experience, Health Policy Politics, YouTube https://www.youtube.com/watch?v=1Y4ubyz3fbY (Accessed 19 February 2024)
2. Regan S., Understanding the Dark Night of the Soul (+ How to Get Through it), mgbmindfulness https://www.mindbodygreen.com/articles/dark-night-of-soul (Accessed 4 May 2024)
3. Descartes R., Discourse on Method, 1637, Britannica https://www.britannica.com/topic/cogito-ergo-sum (Accessed 4 May 2024)

WHERE ARE YOU GOING?

As I stood before the group as the leader in that laughter yoga class, reality hit me hard in the face like WTF! **I'd thought it was where I was going and had felt sure I was on the right track.**

But I wasn't!

My master's degree dissertation researched the use of humour in therapy and, not only was I passionate about it, but I believed it and laughter were my way forward.

So, at fifty-one, I went off to America to attend a big humour conference (only in America) after which I trained there as a laughter yoga teacher.

Yeeehaaa!

The taster sessions I organised when I got back home were well attended, but no one was willing to pay for a class. Each time I offered a session or series of sessions with a fee, nothing.

Not even the sound of crickets!

It was in that last free session that I realised I'd got it all wrong yet right at the same time.

The whole point of laughter yoga is to induce laughter in people so they can reap the benefits of it. And there are many.[1]

But, as I was leading the group in revving up laughter sounds, a visual-feeling-reeling flashback hit me of my mother, grandmother, and a female cousin laughing hysterically.

They seemed to trigger each other into more uncontrolled laughter at each laugh, rolling about physically in the cacophony of high-pitched shrieking, yelling, and even drooling at times.

A cameo of the emotional instability rife in my family.

Instantly, I recognised how terrified I'd been as a child being around that very unsafe, unstable energy.

There was craziness and traumatisation to be worked with for me to heal and grow.

So, while the laughter yoga never lifted off as an income, it showed me the therapeutic work I desperately needed to clear a whole load of "stuff" that had crippled me in relationships.

Now, if you're standing at the Every-Which-Way Signpost, lost in the Wilderness, or Adrift Without a Rudder, you'd be forgiven for thinking that what you want to know is where you're going 100% guaranteed.

I get it and that can happen.

However, where you think you're going could lead you to an unexpected "something" that will be more aligned with your highest and greatest good. Even if you don't think it is!

A question… How do you make God laugh?

The answer is… Show her your plans!

Remember, we create plans to make an uncertain world feel as if it is certain.

However, Mark Batterson, an American Pastor, suggests **the Divine has her own plan for you even if you have one already in place.** And, if your plan is not aligned with the Divine's plan, by hook or by crook, whatever you do, it's the Divine's plan that will unfold.[2]

Just as it did with me!

The humour trail didn't work out as I envisaged. Instead, it was a vehicle through which the Divine got me to do the crucial work I needed to develop healthy relationships.

I know!

It's a human and a logical mind thing to want certainty. In reality, there is none.

Only this moment, and this moment, and this moment, and so on, where, in fact, anything might happen from winning the lottery to losing your job.

The only certainty is uncertainty!

But here's the thing. That doesn't mean you can't be guided in a particular direction. And to receive that direction, you can limber up with the "If you could be or do anything in the world, what would that be?" question.

Write yourself a long list of answers. Don't censor them even if you think what you write is ridiculous.

This exercise is designed to tap into your Wild Soul's design as well as the Divine's plan for you, so go wild!

Your logical mind is bound to find some stuff strange so thank it for its opinion if it interrupts... and then continue.

Sit quietly and go for it. Write a list as fast as you can of all the things you could be and do, including the bizarre.

Go high, broad, deep, round the corner, upside down, diagonally and horizontally, sideways on, back to front and, I have to say it, every which way in your answers.

Let answers trigger other answers.

Riff with the Universe and beyond.

When you think you're finished, close your eyes, take three deep breaths, and see what else your hand wants to write.

When you are truly cooked, read through swiftly, and ring the top three that your eye and hand want to ring, even if they're bizarre.

Remember my story about wanting to be a clinical psychologist and the disillusionment that led me to become a psychotherapist?

Both occupations have a "wanting to help people in a particular way" theme.

Where you're going will have a theme too.

So, soften your eyes' gaze, gently notice what lies in your peripheral vision... Then invite yourself to write down the theme that connects your top three answers.

Even if the theme sounds barmy there will be a nugget of truth in it somewhere.

If you get nothing, make your best guess because guesses hold magic in them. Very often they have at their heart what is!

Finally, let your eye and hand be attracted to #1 of your top three answers, and ring it heavily.

Together with your theme, if you have one, this is the working hypothesis of where you're going as we explore next how you might do that very human thing of tripping yourself up.

When have you thought you knew where you were going only to have an unexpected "something" redirect you?

How do you feel about your theme and working hypothesis?

Did anything in this section surprise you and if so, why?

Where are you now on the Treasure Map?

ENDNOTES

1. Busby M., Why the health benefits of laughter yoga make you smile, *The Guardian* online 9 October 2022 https://www.theguardian.com/lifeandstyle/2022/oct/09/why-the-health-benefits-of-laughter-yoga-will-make-you-smile
2. Batterson, M., *Soulprint: Discovering Your Divine Destiny*, 2011, Multnomah Books. Random House Inc., New York.

WHERE MIGHT YOU TRIP YOURSELF UP?

It was all down to my then-husband that I didn't even attend the first meeting to discuss *the possibility* of attending a psychology degree.

Just the possibility.

Nothing more!

Early on in my marriage, the seeds of where I was going and what I came here to do started to emerge when I worked as PA to the head of the humanities faculty in a local college.

By the way, **that was a great move on the part of my Wild Soul to manoeuvre me into a job in higher education**, an area in which I'd never worked before. Immersed in education, my urge to follow the psychology trail surfaced.

By chance, I saw a psychology degree course being offered at Queen Mary's University in London. With my heart in my throat, I courageously wrote to them to see if I was eligible to apply.

My expectations were low, so I was surprised to receive a reply within days. I can't remember what I'd written to them, but I can remember the enthusiastic response to me in their letter.

My heart beat faster and faster as I read they'd love me to come in for a conversation about applying for the degree programme. Then my head and fear kicked in.

I hadn't told my conservative with a small "c" husband I'd written to them.

What would he think? What would he say? Even more, what would his very traditional family say? How would I be able to even do a degree with having to work too?

Remember, we were only at the "come in and let's talk" stage, but suddenly all my fears about being acceptable, liked, and loved, never mind the unconscious varieties of "I'm not good enough," blew up.

So, I wrote back, thanking them for the offer and saying my husband didn't want me to become a student, and, therefore, I wasn't best placed to attend the degree course at that time.

It later proved to be true when I eventually attended another psychology degree course. Not only did he absolutely not like me doing it, he passive-aggressively avoided supporting me.

I remember him saying I should have done it before I got married. However, by then I had more self-belief and gumption than I had during the Queen Mary's episode.

What I'd done then was to use my husband as an excuse for not exploring the possibility of doing what I desired.

With hindsight, I saw the real reason was me being shit scared to do it for all kinds of reasons, including a lack of belief in myself.

That's how I tripped myself up with a plethora of fears.

Deeper, under the general fears, there's usually one about succeeding (me putting my head above the parapet equals getting shot down equals humiliation and shame) **which can be more ferocious than the fear of failing** (looking a fool and another kind of humiliation and shame).

Sometimes there seem to be outside circumstances that trip you up or hold you back from where you're going. But please double-check you're not using them as excuses to not go where you're going, just like I did.

Be freakin' honest with yourself.

Acknowledge it's an excuse and consciously choose to hold yourself back, if that's what you're doing, because...

You can never disidentify from something you've not already identified with.

So, by acknowledging you've put yourself on the Great Wall of Self-sabotage or have taken a trip into Anti-life Gremlins Land, you've opened up the choice to do something different. To go where you're going whatever's going on!

Sometimes you can achieve what you desire without a hitch and sometimes it seems as though nothing's working for you. Frustration and beating your head against a brick wall can feel familiar.

Again, check exactly what's going on.

Sit with your Wild Soul's inner wisdom by closing your eyes, taking a few deep and slow breaths, and focusing deep down in your belly.

Then ask, "What's getting in my way right now?"

Take whatever it gives you, asking questions for clarification if need be.

If it's a fear, imagine the part of you that is fearful, and converse with it so you can understand it better. You're then more able to give it what it needs for its health and growth.

Remember that Love and fear can't coexist and use the mantra, "I forgive myself for feeling fear and choose Love instead."

Finally, it's very human to have fear tripping you up.

Every time you challenge yourself to grow, develop, and evolve into more of who you were designed to be, **it's likely you'll feel fear because you're going into the freakin' unknown.**

Remember, we crave certainty, and there's nothing certain about the unknown.

Will they still love me? Will they approve of what I'm doing? What if they don't like me going where I'm going? Ya-di-ya-di-ya-di-ya!

So here's a tale to inspire courage in you, mon brave...

A cousin of mine who had been a ward sister was studying to be a doctor. BTW, she was married with four young children which must have been a logistical nightmare.

In year three or four of her seven-year medical degree, disaster struck. Her husband's business folded, there was no money, and their home was repossessed.

Did she throw in the towel?

No, she did not!

The family moved into a friend's small and empty house, he got work of some kind, and she successfully continued with her degree and the logistical nightmare of four young children.

Where there is a Will there is always but always a way.
Similarly, there's always at least one resource to overcome the tripping up!

When have you tripped yourself up in life?

What's the main fear that trips you up?

Feel the fear and repeat at least three times, "I forgive myself for feeling the fear of (e.g. success, failure, humiliation) and choose love instead!"

What changes?

Where are you now on the Treasure Map?

WHERE IS THE RESOURCE TO OVERCOME YOUR "TRIP UP"?

When my then husband finally fessed up to me he'd built up big business debts he couldn't pay, I was as frightened as hell. I wasn't earning much. Certainly not enough to cover maintaining a home, us, and two children.

My long-time fears of ending up as a bag lady blew up in technicolour, particularly as he had absolutely no plan B.

However, after a few days of oh-shit-oh-shit-oh-shit-oh-shit, I decided to clear the house of anything we hadn't used in twelve months and take it to a car boot sale.

Unbelievably, I cleared over £100 which was a lot of money back in the day.

He took over the car boot sale venture and we eventually downsized our house at £0, nothing saved but with nothing left owing.

A definite result!

When I look at what I did there and compare it with my shorthand-and-typing venture when my son's father was leaving us, **I recognise my biggest resources were resilience and resourcefulness with a good shot of courage.**

Different circumstances but the same resources helped me overcome major examples of external life circumstances tripping me up.

And the biggest resource of all is the ability to take action!

Remember, the Spark of your Wild Soul I wrote about in "You are more than your personality"? It's the aspect of you that can observe non-judgementally what's going on and, through the power of Will, can spur you into action.

The word "Will" is often associated with oppression and exploitation. But *your* Will, your ability to make decisions and act upon them, is the complete opposite.

The Will's three qualities, strong, skilful, and good, if engaged, help ensure you do what needs to be done effectively for the highest good of yourself and others.

Whether your "tripper-uppers" are external or internal, your use of Will to create overcoming action is essential.

What about self-sabotage, when *internal* factors tripped me up? These have mostly been fears with a dollop of I'm not good enough in its various forms thrown into the mix.

When I've looked at the internal causes of tripping myself up, I don't come quickly to a remedy.

So, I've taken action and used my Will to engage in therapeutic work to undo limiting beliefs and resolve childhood fears. Internal resources like curiosity and persistence definitely help there!

Of course, there are external practical resources that help. Just as learning shorthand and typing was essential to improve my job marketability as a young woman. And car boot sales were a perfect resource to raise much-needed cash. However...

I'm purposely focusing here on internal resources so you can realise you're far more resourceful than you think in overcoming whatever trips you up.

You could call these internal resources personality characteristics or "values". I see them as emanating from a higher level, that they are, in fact, **spiritual qualities and resources for "being".**[1]

Now, having identified some self-tripper-uppers in the previous section, let yourself reflect on earlier periods in your life when you've faced difficult times.

They might have a similar theme or have no connection. It doesn't matter. Journal whatever comes up, letting your inner wisdom provide them for you.

When you have at least two self-tripper-uppers, **ask your inner wisdom for the resource or resources, the spiritual qualities of being, that helped you get through or overcome tripping yourself up.**

Journal whatever you get as you'll work with them a little later. But first...

When I was nearly fifty I had a reoccurrence of an earlier problem with a slipped disc in my spine. If you think of the pain as a permanent raging toothache or never-ending labour, you'll get what I was going through.

Anyhow, I was recovering but feeling incredibly unsafe. Bag lady fears reared their head plus fears about my physical being. Would I ever get back to my normal activity level again?

A friend suggested I use the mantra, "Right now I'm safe," while I was taking my medicinal short walks around my local park.

I was very sceptical about mantras, affirmations, and those things I saw as "space-cadet-love-and-light" bullshit at the time. However, I decided to give it a go.

Oh, how boring it was to repeat the mantra at first!

I souped it up with the addition of "absolutely." "Right now I am absolutely safe."

Mmm... A bit more oomph to it but it still felt mechanical and boring.

I am so glad I persevered.

One day in my third mantra week, I was walking around the park repeating the mantra as if my life depended on it when SHAZAM! I was stopped in my tracks by the realisation I actually did feel safe!

I thought, "This shit works!"

Ever since, I've been an advocate of using mantras to shift from unproductive to creative thoughts, feelings, and beliefs.

But you won't catch me chanting in a month of Sundays!

So give it a go yourself.

Create a right-now-I'm-absolutely-xyz mantra. Xyz is the resource/s you need to overcome what might trip you up.

If it's courage, you're courageous. If it's peace, you're peaceful. If it's love, you're loved.

And, if it's all three resources, it's, "Right now, I'm absolutely courageous, peaceful, and loved."

Choose to repeat your mantra every day with a particular activity that lasts at least 10 minutes. Could be travelling to work or a journey on public transport, walking, doing the washing up... Whatever.

Prepare to be surprised and delighted when, about the three-week mark, you notice the resource or resources you needed have changed how you feel and behave.

You will have actually embodied that spiritual quality.

Positive energy taken in repeatedly will always result in a positive outcome, in this case how you feel.

Another way to look at what's happened is that you've re-programmed your brain. It hears the spiritual qualities you want to develop, rubs its hands together in glee and says, "You want more of xyz? I'm on it!"

These spiritual qualities not only help you overcome how you might trip yourself up from getting where you're going, but they'll also support what you came here to do!

> Do you recognise any repeating patterns in your self-tripping-up?
>
> Using the spiritual qualities you identified that helped you get through or overcome tripping yourself up, where else in your life could they help you?
>
> Did anything in this section surprise you and, if so, why?
>
> Where are you now on the Treasure Map?

IMPORTANT NB. If you want to scream because you think this whole WHERE YOU'RE GOING section hasn't worked for you, please be aware that it has worked even if it doesn't seem like it.

You will have exercised all the psycho-spiritual muscles you need to move forward, and your unconscious is working the material churned up to get you ready for the next section, WHAT DID YOU COME HERE TO DO?

So, go do it, magnificent women. And, when you have, you might or might not need to revisit this section with the information you'll then know.

ENDNOTES

1. Access the "What Are Your Spiritual Qualities?" PDF at www.re-discovered-life

4 WHAT DID YOU COME HERE TO DO?

YOUR MISSION ON EARTH, PURPOSE, AND MEANING

"WTF is that?"

I'm sitting in the training room with my student peers in the middle of a guided imagery exercise about our spiritual purpose for being born. With my eyes shut, I hear the trainer's voice move the exercise towards its completion. But my logical mind and personality are in overdrive.

"Trust you to have such a crazy purpose!"

"What the feck does it mean?"

"I'm going to look so stupid when we share our purposes!"

And so it was.

As we went around the seated circle, one by one they shared their purpose, all sounding perfectly intelligible until it got to me.

They'd clearly reached Clarity Castle while I was most definitely in WTF Quick Sand.

There was nothing for it but to say it.

"The birthing of humanity for the birthing of humanity."

No comment was made about anyone's purpose, but it felt to me as if the lack of comment about mine just proved what a shitty one it was. And my peers were probably all laughing behind their polite, listening faces.

Until I reminded myself I have a crazy psyche.

For example, when we were guided to draw a picture of our Wild Souls in another training module, my peers drew butterflies, beautiful and bountiful gardens, and awesome birds of flight.

Me?

My image was the shaving you get when you sharpen a pencil!

You know how it curls round and round as you turn the pencil?

It was only later that I realised it was a symbol for the eternal spiral so gorgeously illustrated in the lines of our DNA and the cyclical, spiralling nature of our growth.

It's also about simplicity which is the numero uno spiritual quality in my work, how I learn the best, and how I teach.

Having remembered my pencil shaving, I shifted from self-abusive criticism and comparisonitis to just sitting with the seemingly bizarre purpose of "the birthing of humanity for the birthing of humanity."

Just sitting and waiting to see where it went. Some days later, in the shower, I suddenly realised what it meant.

Insights often come when you least expect them, so it's imperative you record them.

You think you'll remember, but, I promise you, you won't.

So, dripping water, I rushed to my study and wrote, "The birthing of humanity for the birthing of humanity.

It's me... It's freakin' me!

I'm being asked to work on myself, to free my humanity, who I am at essence, from all the crap conditioning that occludes it. The better I might work with someone else to uncover their own humanity!"

In that moment, my life had a purpose that gave it meaning. I had a reason for living and experienced myself and life as worthwhile.

Life wasn't all about birth, death, and the bit between but was about much more.

So, *that* was my mission on Earth!

I wrote earlier about your body being a spacesuit to carry your Wild Soul.

And, just like an astronaut arriving on the moon, imagine that you landed on Earth with a mission to fulfil; your purpose for being here. **A mission that only you can fulfil in the unique way you can fulfil it.**

There's a mistaken belief that your purpose is something specific like feeding the poor in a xyz country.

But your mission on Earth is never a thing. It's always a theme.

Just like my "the birthing of humanity for the birthing of humanity." It's a theme which could be expressed in many ways.

For example, rather than become a spiritual psychotherapist coach, I could fulfil my mission by being an aromatherapist, a positive psychology trainer, a pop star, a leadership coach, an inspirational card writer, or even a car mechanic.

Or, in a serial career, I could, of course, manifest my mission on Earth through all of them. Although I suspect being a pop star would be a bit of a stretch!

However, you could already be doing something which unconsciously you've been inspired to do because of your mission whether you're aware of it or not.

It's the thing that you're passionate about, that gives meaning to you and your life.

There's a story that went the rounds on social media some years ago, so I don't know whether it's true or not. But it was about a son who had learning difficulties and worked as a bag packer at a supermarket checkout.

He noticed so many people seemed to be in low spirits and wanted to do something to help lift them. With the help of his dad, he downloaded inspirational quotations, cut each into a thin strip, and popped one into each bag he packed.

It wasn't long before he became known for what he was doing. And, because of the positive effect it had, the queue at whatever checkout he was working would be the longest and most cheerful in the whole supermarket.

His mission seems to have had something to do with spreading happiness!

When pondering your mission, the most important thing is to avoid a full-frontal attack on your Wild Soul which, as the holder of your original design, is the keeper of your "mission on Earth" information.

So, no heavy-duty intellectual or analytical exploration as it pisses your Wild Soul right off and it retreats at a fast rate of knots. Instead...

Come at finding your mission on Earth left field and sideways.

It helps loosen things up a bit by writing a list of everything you love or have loved being or doing right from when you can first remember up to the present day.

Spread the writing over a few days as you might well remember something stimulated by your previous writing.

Then, trusting your eyes and hand, as you've done previously, circle the top three most attractive things on your list and see if there's a shared theme.

If you don't see a theme, no problem.

Be easy with it.

No straining or mental fandangos.

Trust your inner wisdom and adopt an attitude of curiosity.

You might also like to visit your Beautiful Safe Meadow as you did in "Imagination and a resource for your adventure" earlier in RE-DISCOVERED. If you do, just invite your Wild Soul to join you and let it show you or tell you the theme of your mission here on Earth.

Take whatever you get however bizarre!

All will unfold as it needs to unfold.

Remember that I heard mine. You might see yours, feel it in your body, or sense it in some other way. And while its meaning might be straightforward, sometimes, like mine, it most definitely is not!

Lastly, if you get nothing, please, please honour the "nothing".

We each have our own rhythms with rediscovery and it might just mean yours is in the delicious marinating process and not yet ready to be revealed.

Over the days, weeks, or months to come you will realise your mission on Earth. It might be through seeing a message on a billboard, a song you hear, or a film you're watching.

Anything but anything in this world or beyond could be the trigger that reveals your particular mission here on Earth.

Even reading the next section about your spiritual fingerprint could do it.

Stay open. Be curious. And chill!

> Who are the top three people you most admire and why?
>
> What do they all have in common?
>
> What do your previous two answers tell you about your mission on Earth?
>
> Where are you now on the Treasure Map?

YOUR SPIRITUAL FINGERPRINT

When my children got to a certain age, I told them both that if they ever needed therapy I would pay for it. For the life of me, I can't remember why, but my guess is I was all too aware of how my behaviour might have screwed them up and wanted to make amends.

Anyhow, my daughter took me up on my offer in no uncertain terms. Being a psychotherapist, I knew not to ask her about the details of the therapy, but, at some point, I asked her how it was going in a general sort of way.

She remarked that her woman therapist wasn't warm and mumsy like me!

I laughed at the idea I was warm and mumsy, but, remember, this is the child who'd overheard my telephone conversations with prospective clients, friends, and family over the years.

And that got me thinking about archetypes.

Archetypes are universal templates of people, behaviours, and personalities that can influence human behaviour.[1]

Carl Jung, a Swiss psychiatrist, suggested, "Archetypes symbolise basic human motivations, values, and personalities."[2]

We all have an understanding of what the Mother template would look like.

You had to have a mother to be born. And you'll have had surrogate "mothers" in the form of friends, relatives, or strangers who've treated you in a way you would call motherly.

For each archetype, there's universal understanding of what it means to embody it.

Think of the Orphan, the Angel, the Magician, the Rebel, the Wise Woman aka Witch... You get an immediate sense of the characteristics belonging to each of them.

You also never have just one archetype but a mixture of several. For example, I recognise embodying, among others, the Mother, the Crone, the Witch, and have to watch out not to act out the Controller.

Oh yes... There are times!

I believe the archetypes with which you identify form part of your spiritual fingerprint.

Remember my #1 spiritual value in my work is Love which fits rather well with the Mother. Not so good with the Controller though!

I also believe the spiritual qualities with which we most identify form part of our spiritual fingerprint.

For example, if I carry Love in my spiritual fingerprint, I'm bound to have a different spiritual fingerprint from someone who exhibits meanness and aggression. My spiritual fingerprint, the energy I emit out into the world, will have a different vibe.

Your fingerprint influences your relationships too.

My ex-husband was always critical of me for getting involved in conversations with strangers when we were out together. I suspect it got up his nose that my warmth was met by warmth from others.

The scientist in me would say surely that's about having different personality characteristics.

Well, yes, I was gregarious and he was not, but ultimately personality characteristics also arise from the archetypes with which you identify.

And, as you might have guessed…

The bottom line in our spiritual fingerprint is the extent to which we identify with and express the divine healing energy of Love.

Also known as the glue that holds the Universe together and, potentially, everything else too.

Martin Buber, a twentieth-century philosopher, proposed two kinds of relationship encounters, one without the presence of Love and one with its presence.[3]

He called the first I/It where you see the other as an "it" whom you can use for your benefit in some way.

What's in it for me?

This type of relationship is exemplified by old-fashioned sales techniques where the only point of the other human being was to get them to buy whatever you were selling.

Love?

Nowhere to be seen.

The second kind of relationship he called I/Thou.

Immediately, just with the word "thou", you'll intimate this relationship is a very different kettle of fish.

In I/Thou encounters there's a connection of one Wild Soul with another, recognising the essential sacredness of each other.

Indeed, Love fuels this encounter where the question is not "What's in it for me?" but "How can I be of service to you?"

When I think of I/Thou it also reminds me of the Sanskrit word "Namaste." The word means I bow to you, a gesture of respect and gratitude for the Divine in others as it is in yourself.

A recognition of Wild Soul-ness!

Buber suggests that relationship is what gives meaning to your life. That relationship is part of what you came here to do.

It seems to me how much you have or don't have the capacity for an I/Thou relationship is part of your spiritual fingerprint too.

Being available for an I/Thou relationship doesn't mean you accept unfair treatment, abuse, undermining, or any other mistreatment meted out by people who are still unconsciously asleep.

And it doesn't mean you have to turn the other cheek, either!

It does mean you align your integrity with Love in all you say and do in the world. As Mahatma Gandhi encouraged us, "Be the change you wish to see in the world."

Do I screw up sometimes?

You bet I do, and, you know what, having a good gossip and dishing the dirt feels quite liberating when you have a history of being a "good girl". But it most definitely isn't loving.

What am I going to do?

Beat myself up?

No!

What I do is have compassion for my not-so-great personality part involved in dishing the dirt. And more frequently make choices on the side of my spiritual fingerprint whenever I can.

And here's the thing...

The energy we put out is most definitely the energy we get back.

Archetypes for the greater good, the Divine, the healing energy of Love, and I/Thou relationships are the best you can carry and offer.

For your spiritual fingerprint is, indeed, part of your mission here on Earth!

> What archetypes do you embody?
>
> Imagine having an I/It encounter and then an I/Thou encounter and notice how you feel in each case.
>
> What does your spiritual fingerprint tell you about what you came here to be and do?
>
> Where are you now on the Treasure Map?

ENDNOTES

1. Access the "What Are Your Archetypes?" PDF at www.re-discovered-life
2. Cherry K., MSEd, What are the Jungian Archetypes, updated 5 May 2024, verywellmind.com, https://www.verywellmind.com/what-are-jungs-4-major-archetypes-2795439#toc-the-origins-of-jungian-archetypes (Accessed 9 June 2024)
3. Buber M., *I and Thou*, 1970, Simon and Schuster

YOUR MISSION ON EARTH, PURPOSE, AND MEANING REVISITED

Before I knew my mission on Earth, I knew something was missing but I didn't know what.

In fact, I knew more about what I didn't want to have, be, and do. That included trying to be a respectable, suburban semi-detached wife and mother including Chair of the PTA.

I tried. I promise you.

I really tried, but, while it seemed purposeful, I was slowly dying inside.

No wonder I suffered from depression during those years. I had to depress myself, who I really am, to get into that constricted respectable box.

I spent a lot of time in Fear Central, the Stuck Bog, Bloody Burnout, the Wilderness, the Doldrums, and the Great Wall of Self-sabotage not to mention wandering in the Desert.

Just recently, I found some photographs of myself during the pre-knowing-my-mission-on-Earth-time and I had the deadest eyes you can imagine. Indeed, I see myself then as "living dead".

Apart from my children, there was little that touched my heart, my being, or my soul.

However, I'd done a Psychology A level, and that stirred my desire to help people, and the idea of being a clinical psychologist came to me as the way forward. So, I followed the route to become that.

You know the rest!

But the nub of the story is I followed the "clues".

That reminds me of an old saying, "Let go and let God". Reframe God to the Universe, Shera, or any other universal benevolent creative energy that feels right for you.

And the clues I chose to follow came at me in divine order...

If I hadn't done the Psychology A level...

I wouldn't have met the student on the degree course who told me about the spiritual psychotherapy programme,

and if I hadn't trained for seven years in that programme,

I wouldn't have found my mission on Earth and, fast forward over forty years,

I wouldn't still be living a life with meaning and purpose.

BUT...

I didn't discover my mission on Earth, what I came here to do, in one leap even though it might sound as if I did!

If you got a sense of what you came here to do, congratulations. Let it marinate for a while. At the same time, watch out for clues to help you decide how you'll manifest your mission here on Earth.

If you didn't get a sense of what you came here to do, congratulations! You're in exactly the right place according to the Divine and your Wild Soul.

What that means is there's more to this particular adventure for you. So, check out with your inner wisdom what to be or do next.

For example, you might be asked to stay still, and do nothing. To let the muddy waters take the time they need to clear without an intervention from you.

You might be guided to go about your everyday business and wait for the sign that reveals your mission on Earth.

Remember it can be as bizarre as seeing a particular interaction between two people or the name of a book you see in a shop window.

Timing is all.

You might be urged to return to the exercises you've done in this section to open your eyes to what you didn't see the first time, or to restimulate the mission-on-Earth-juices.

OR…

Having read everything up to now, make one huge freakin' guess as to what you came here for!

The Divine likes a big ask, so make your guess huge. Dive into the realms of what feels impossible and see what turns up.

Remember my "the birthing of humanity for the birthing of humanity" and how weird that was?

Let the poet in you wax lyrical, the dreamer in you outdo itself, the artist in you paint a million colours and the magician in you erect 100 golden rings in a circle in the flickering of an eye… SHAZAM!

Just be open to whatever information you get however it lands!

Alternatively, if you know what your mission on Earth is, or have made a humongous guess, or still have no idea…

How would you love to manifest as yourself right now?

Yes, even if you have no idea!

Remember, I wanted "the thing", to be a clinical psychologist. And that "thing" took me on an adventure during which I eventually found my life's mission, my purpose.

If you're called to do so, go back to the section "WHERE ARE YOU GOING?" and see how it's been refined through knowing what you know now.

AND, finally…

Do not get precious about knowing your mission on Earth.

I'm sure you'll be expressing it in your life somehow because that's what we do. Hiding it, as it were, in plain sight!

I've been known to say to a client that their purpose right now was RE-COVERY from depression, bereavement, relationship breakdown, or whatever they've come for the healing.

Just as your purpose right now, if nothing else, is most certainly re-discovering yourself.

Indeed, taking the RE-DISCOVERED adventure is just one of the ways you can express your sacred mission on Earth right here, right now!

> What's changed for you through reading this section?
>
> How does RE-DISCOVERED sit with you as your purpose right now?
>
> AND, if you know your mission on Earth yet or not, what meaning would you love to have for your life?
>
> (The last question gives you one of those clues I wrote about!)
>
> Where are you now on the Treasure Map?

5 THE END

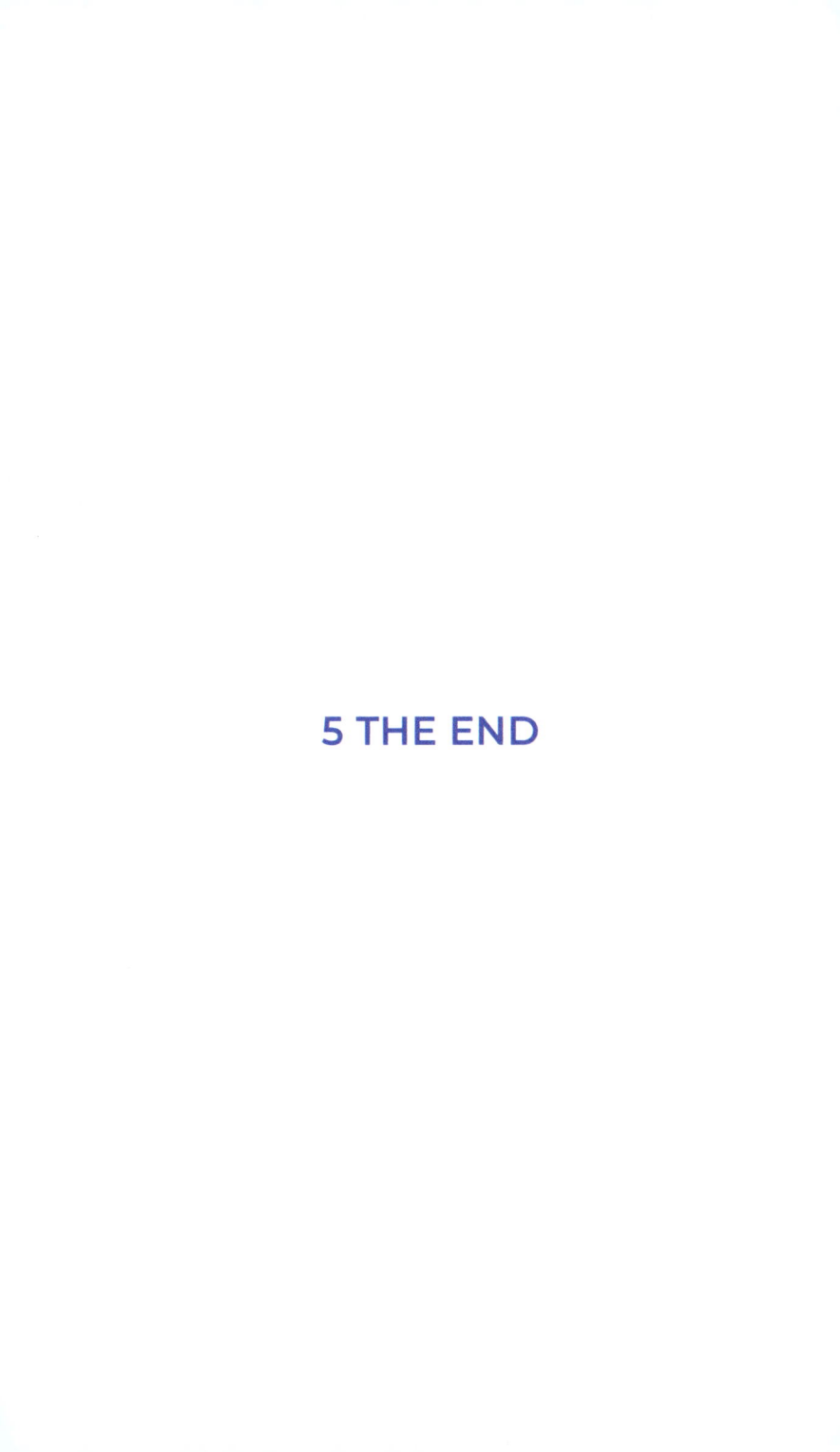

CHOICE OR NO CHOICE

Paradoxically, I prevaricated heavily when it came to writing this section.

Shall I write this? Shall I write that? Or would it be better to go there? Or there?

You know how it is when you can't get a handle on something and your mind drives you bonkers with alternatives.

Until I laughed out loud and told myself to just start writing, do the thing, and see what comes.

Just CHOOSE to do something rather than encourage the freakin' inertia prevarication creates.

Taking action is always key.

Not choosing is still unconsciously choosing by omission, so why not go for it however it turns out?

Remember my wedding day? My Wild Soul was yelling at me not to go ahead. Perhaps it knew my marriage would be a detour. Who knows?

What I do know is, despite the warning, I chose to go ahead.

Why?

Because I could.

Because I, like all other human beings, have free will to choose what I do or do not do.

The problem is we often make our choices through conditioned lenses based on what we've learned is acceptable or not, what's appropriate or not, and what significant others think is right or not right for us.

So free will isn't that free after all!

However, the thing is...

If you choose Adventure A, you'll go down the Adventure A learning path.

If you choose Adventure B, you'll go down the Adventure B learning path.

And so on...

What you then do with what you've chosen to do is also down to you.

I suspect if I'd stayed in the marriage, my life would have continued down the depression slippery slope until... Well, perhaps I would have eventually succeeded in taking my life.

But, hey, in my forties I chose to end the marriage. I just couldn't face the years ahead being with someone so wrong for me, as I was for him.

At the same time, the unhappy marriage didn't stop me from following my Wild Soul's inner wisdom. It steered me closer and closer to fulfilling my mission on Earth and choosing a way to manifest it that worked for me.

When that happens...

It feels like the penny's dropped or a key has fitted into a lock so sweetly it's almost sexy!

You feel it as your heart's desire, your passion, and nothing but nothing will get in your way except, perhaps, you, as we explored in the "Where might you trip yourself up?" section.

So, at some unconscious level, I'd made a choice aligned with my original design, and, despite the seeming error of my marriage, it was shit or bust toward fulfilling my mission on Earth.

You've made some choices through the adventure of reading RE-DISCOVERED. I've encouraged you to make them in ways that discourage interference by your logical mind and conditioning.

That makes them more likely to be choices in line with your original design. But even if something went wrong and they're not, like my training as a laughter yoga teacher, it's not the end of the world.

Whatever choices you've made take you on a valuable learning adventure for your personal and spiritual growth.

Ultimately that will feed into your mission on Earth, even if it's about how not to embody and manifest it in the world!

Because, your personal and spiritual growth is a funny and curious thing, as I'll also be telling the management if I'm able!

> Think of a time when you made a choice that didn't work out as you hoped and write down what you learned from it.
>
> Think of a time when you made a choice and it did work out as you hoped and write down what you learned from it.
>
> Think of a time when you failed to make a choice and write down what you learned from that.
>
> What do your answers tell you?
>
> (I rest my case! Whatever you do or don't do leads to evolutionary learning IF you're open to it.)
>
> Where are you now on the Treasure Map?

EVOLUTION AND THE SHAPE OF IT

What's true about personal and spiritual growth is you often only realise you've evolved with hindsight.

It seeps into your consciousness, "Well, look at that. I'm not being defensive when someone challenges me anymore!"

Well, until the next time it crops up.

There's a handed-down story about a man who walks down a road with a freakin' big hole in it. Only he doesn't see the hole and falls right in.

The next time he walks down the same road he knows there's a freakin' big hole but can't seem to help himself and, once again, falls right in.

And the next time he walks down the same road he's aware of the hole and chooses to walk safely around it.

Yeeehaaa!

Only, the next time he walks down that road, he doesn't see the hole and falls right in once again.

The RE-DISCOVERED adventure, hopefully, will have helped you recognise yourself falling into some holes too, some of which you might now navigate more safely.

So why on earth would you, like that man, not see them again?

Oh, if it was only that easy!

The nature of personal and spiritual evolution is not always linear and progressive onward and upward, but more like a spiral.

Think of pinecones, curly hair, snail shells, our DNA, and even galaxies. They're all spirals. **And it turns out that growing in a spiral is an evolutionary smart way to do it.**[1]

As for being human, you deal with an issue at one turn of the spiral, do some healing, create a more life-affirming belief maybe, change a behaviour or two, and, phew, you think that's done.

Hoo-flippin-ray!

But, hey, you walk down the road again, don't see the whacking great hole and fall right in. It seems like you're back at stage one of that issue.

But you're not!

Where you are is at a higher turn of the spiral.

You're a more evolved and resourceful being and, because of the work you did at the turn of the lower spiral, you're now ready to heal aspects of the issue you couldn't heal then.

Think about feeling discontented, lost, or overwhelmed. I bet this isn't the only time in your life you've experienced those feelings albeit perhaps not as strongly as you have recently.

They've occurred at different stages and times in your life. Only this time your Wild Soul is insisting you pay attention, learn what you're meant to learn and do something about it.

And now, with your current resources, it's a rite of passage that leads you from who you were to rediscovering who you really are, or, at the very least, who you're becoming, where you're going, and what you came here to do.

Job done?

Who knows!

What's important is if, at another turn of the spiral you're called to revisit feeling discontented, lost, or overwhelmed, **RE-DISCOVERED will have given you tools and techniques to get you through the rite of passage.**

I know. It seems like a crazy system. As you know, if there's a place to go when I'm physically dead, I'll be having that word!

You might also be reassured to know there are times when I raise my eyes heavenward and exclaim very loudly to the Divine, "Haven't I done enough?"

The current answer is always NO, and, in its way, that's a blessing!

Richard Bach, the author of the 1970s cult book *Jonathan Livingston Seagull*, proposed a test. If you want to know whether you've fulfilled your mission on Earth, the answer is NO if you're still alive.[2]

So, we're doing good…

There's more to go, more iterations of who you really are, where you're going, and what you came here to be and do as you grow and become the more and more resourceful human being you were designed to be.

> Flick back through your life and notice earlier times of being discontented or lost.
>
> What have you learned this time that you didn't earlier?
>
> What's your biggest learning about the way you evolve?
>
> Where are you now on the Treasure Map?

ENDNOTES

1. Hand E., Patterns in nature: where to spot spirals, 25 April 2019, Science World Online https://www.scienceworld.ca/stories/patterns-nature-where-spot-spirals/ (Accessed 4 May 2024)
2. Bach R., *Jonathan Livingston Seagull: A story*, 2015, Harper Thorsons

Please take 5 minutes to leave me a review, it helps other people to decide if they want to read the book, and I'll be eternally grateful. If you're reading on Kindle just scroll to the end of the book. If you're reading the paperback, please go to your favourite bookstore.

Remember, you can get the promised downloads at www.re-discovered.life or scan the QR code.

REINCARNATION BUT NOT AS YOU KNOW IT!

Some years ago, I developed a block in marketing my work. I would second guess what to say when networking, stumble to find the word, hesitate and generally sound as if the last thing I wanted in the world was to tell you about myself and what I did.

I was working with an energetic intergalactic coach at the time.

Was she really? I don't know but she went to places energetically for which I have no words. And, on this occasion, she told me my issue could be remedied through past-life work.

More of that later...

I was so desperate to untie my tongue that I let her do past-life work and was astonished by where I went.

That was at the bottom of a millpond, crushed by a millstone on my chest and drowning... Obviously!

So that's where I got my fear of drowning from. That's why I avoid being in water deeper than standing depth like the plague.

Who knows?

It's said that the millpond test was intended to see if you were a witch. If you floated you were and if you drowned you were not but the verdict was a bit too late for the "non-witch" by then.

A kind of Middle Age's lose-lose!

Whether that's historical truth or not is irrelevant. All I know is that after that experience and some healing work, I was able to market myself fluently and successfully.

NOW...

Was it a past-life experience or my psyche conjuring up a metaphor that fitted my predicament and aided my healing?

Who knows?

When anybody asks me about past lives, I respond that I've been reincarnated so many times in this life, that it's more than enough to cope with.

Once, when my very grown-up daughter and I were going through old photos, I remember her stopping at one of herself as a toddler. She remarked how it felt like she was looking at a different person.

If you don't believe you've not been the same person all your life, look at a photograph of you taken 10 years ago, 20 years ago, 30 years ago, or when you were a toddler.

How connected do you feel with that person in the photograph? 100%, 75%, 50%, 25% or 0%?

That's because you've been reincarnating in your own lifetime.

While your Wild Soul remains constant (or not, but for our purposes we don't have to go there), your spacesuit, body, and aspects of your personality get reborn as different ways of being in the world.

And if you're reading RE-DISCOVERED, that's not going to stop because, clearly, you're a growthful person.

On the other hand, some people seem not to change over time and some of them even boast about it. "I'm the same person as I was at 20!"

Goddess forbid… There's no way I'd want to be the same as I was back then. Would you?

But then, what do I know?

Obviously, nothing about what those people came to be and do or, indeed, their mission on Earth. It's a possibility that however little they've changed is exactly what was asked of them by the Divine and their own Wild Soul.

Anyhow, reincarnation is generally seen as the rebirth of the soul in a new body. Or coming back in another form, like a caterpillar or pig, depending on how well you did in this life.

I'm proposing something different.

I propose that in this lifetime you evolve through incarnation and become a variation on a theme time and time again.

How exciting is it to know that you can create iterations of yourself over time that progressively reflect more of who you really are, where you're going, and what you came here to be and do?

Using ideas and practices you've learned in RE-DISCOVERED you can become more and more of your original design.

More of the magnificent woman you are with metaphorical and uber-glorious bells on!

Reflect on who and where you were before you began reading RE-DISCOVERED.

Reflect on who and where you are having read the bulk of RE-DISCOVERED.

What changes do you notice in yourself?

And, for the very last time, where are you now on the Treasure Map?

WHAT'S NEXT?

There's a story about a young violinist. She was new to New York City and was late for a special audition.

Although near the prestigious audition venue she was acutely aware the clock was ticking. So to be sure she hailed a yellow cab and asked the driver if he would tell her the way to get to Carnegie Hall.

He took a minute, looked at her wryly, and replied as only a yellow cab driver would, "Practise, practise, practise!"

And that's what comes next.

Practising all you've learned from RE-DISCOVERED, putting it out there in your everyday life, being more aligned with who you really are, where you're going, and what you came here to do.

Practise until it becomes second nature to you and you feel the "click" of being so comfortable with yourself that it feels like paradise.

Until?

Until the next time you feel discontented or lost.

There's an old rabbinic saying that each blade of grass has an angel whispering to it, "Grow, grow, grow!"

In your case, the whisperer is your glorious Wild Soul.

So, when your inner wisdom urges it, return to reread and work through RE-DISCOVERED again.

Then, at each turn of your growth spiral, you'll read something differently, have a new insight, or realise something about yourself you've not done before.

And so your awesome personal and spiritual evolution continues, expressing more of the magnificent, divine, and precious woman you are!

6 THE END... HONESTLY!

As mentioned in The Treasure Map section at the beginning of RE-DISCOVERED, there's no X marks the spot for the treasure.

And, if you haven't guessed already, that's entirely because the treasure is you, magnificent woman.

The treasure is YOU!

THE LAST WORD

Sarah smiled as she lifted the cup of her favourite coffee, savouring the aroma.

It was a warm summer's day with a gentle breeze as she sat in her small but nourishing garden. She'd made it a cameo of nature that evoked a long deep sigh as her feelings, body, mind, and everything else relaxed.

She reflected that nothing much had changed in her life.

She was still a professional businesswoman. She was still with her logically minded partner and connected to her family and friends.

But as she thought of her relationships, she chuckled.

Her partner had initially been bemused by her request to talk more about what mattered to them. She remembered their initial discomfort but, over time, more meaningful communication had brought them closer.

She was more selective now about which of her family and friends she saw, when she saw them, and what they did together. This too had deepened some relationships although a few had naturally drifted away.

"It is what it is," she thought.

Her material life continued to be a good one. And as she reflected on her latest holiday, the comfort of her home, and the lifestyle she and her partner enjoyed, her eyes pricked with tears.

She felt grateful and blessed.

Still enjoying the same interests, she'd spread her wings by attending a creative writing course. Tentative at first, she was now more confident in expressing herself and had even written some poetry.

Sarah smiled again, a big joyful one, realising she experienced herself and her life more meaningfully than back in those dark days of discontent that led to feeling lost, anxious, and overwhelmed.

That didn't mean things never went wrong, difficulties didn't arise, or she never felt low.

What it did mean was that, fortified by her deep connection to her Wild Soul and inner wisdom, with some personality parts having been integrated, she navigated challenging times more skillfully.

She knew now there was learning, meaning, and purpose in everything!

And then Sarah didn't just smile and she didn't just chuckle. She burst out with rich rolling laughter that scared the birds away…

It wasn't so much that nothing had changed in her life but that everything had changed in her!

THE TREASURE MAP KEY

Each landmark has a brief description and three actions you might or might not take.

As the Taoist philosopher Lao Tzu is credited with asking, "Do you have the patience to wait until muddy water clears itself?"

Just sitting with the place you're at and seeing what emerges from doing nothing is always but always an option...

Adrift Without a Rudder - This is when you're drifting aimlessly with no direction or even the slightest idea of one. You could...

1. Summon up the energy to choose a direction... Any direction!
2. Manifest a paddle of some kind and head for the nearest land.
3. Lie back and whistle, "She'll be coming round the mountain when she comes."

Anti-life Gremlins Land - This is where all your negative and unproductive thoughts and feelings live. They love to come out and bite you on the bum. You could…

1. Attempt to shut them down only to find they get stronger.
2. Acknowledge you've heard them, focus on external reality, and tell them, "Right now, I'm (doing whatever you're doing)" to calm them and centre yourself.
3. Buy yourself some guaranteed against Anti-life Gremlin bum bite trousers!

Bloody Burnout - This is when you've been wiped out by fatigue, frustration, or apathy resulting from prolonged stress, overwork, or intense activity. You could…

1. Focus on recovery with rest, healthy food, and good energy stuff.
2. Drag and force yourself to do whatever you feel duty-bound to do.
3. Dump whatever freakin' caused Bloody Burnout in the first place!

Clear View Mountain Top - This is when you get transported to the top as if by magic and can see the terrain clearly. You could…

1. Feel deeply touched that, out of nowhere, you have connection with both above and below in a sacred moment.

2. Record your experience as a memory prompt so you relive that sacred moment when future inspiration is needed.
3. Job done treat yourself to a cuppa!

Clarity Castle - This is where you have a keen sense of "what is" regarding an event or a situation, including your place in the order of things. You could…

1. Respond accordingly for the greatest good of all involved.
2. Respond accordingly for the greatest good for yourself in particular.
3. Throw up your hands and yell, "Not my circus, not my monkeys."

Desert - Dry and arid, this is where you feel you're surviving rather than thriving and where there's nothing but emptiness and tedium stretching away to all sides of you. You could…

1. Summon up Lawrence of Arabia to evoke fresh eyes with which to experience the Desert.
2. Make for the metaphorical Oasis whose palm trees will shade you, fresh dates will nourish you, and cool water will refresh you.
3. Catch the next "express" camel and get out of there ASAP.

Doing Great Peninsula - This is where you, life, and everything is going swimmingly. You could...

1. Relax into the flow of things and enjoy life moment by moment.
2. Express gratitude and feel blessed that all is well.
3. Get bored and create a drama just for the hell of it!

Doldrums - No wind, no waves. A demotivated and monotonous place of no action or desire for it. You could...

1. Agree with yourself on a set time to 'doldrum' followed by at least one designated action, however small.
2. Read motivational books, like RE-DISCOVERED, to inspire and get you going.
3. Admit defeat, veg out and watch your favourite movie on repeat.

Every-Which-Way Signpost - This is when you see multiple options, but are bamboozled by the choice and don't know which to follow. You could...

1. Close your eyes and point randomly at the signpost with fingers crossed.
2. Take a breath, focus deep down in your belly and ask your inner wisdom which option to take for your highest good.
3. Stand scratching your head and wait for Godot to tell you which to follow. PS Do remember, Godot never comes![1]

Fear Central - This is where you feel fear, even terror, and the anxiety, and overwhelm that comes with it. You could...

1. Breathe deeply and slowly, exhaling more than you take in, to slow down your racing nervous system.
2. Imagine being showered with the healing energy of Love with which fear cannot coexist.
3. Turn fear into fierce by acting as if you are a Sumo wrestler complete with growling loudly as and when.

Great Wall of Self-sabotage - This is what you hit when time and time again you set out to do something and, somehow, always screw it up. You could...

1. STOP and reflectively identify what you're doing or feeling that stops you from achieving your desired outcome.
2. Choose to do and feel the absolute opposite of what you identified.
3. The substantially fortified Great Wall of Self-sabotage is said to be over 21,000 kilometres. Use shedloads of dynamite!

Lake Calm - This is when you're gliding, chilled out, and nothing's fazing you at all whatever's happening in your life. You could...

1. Delight and be fully present in every calm moment by moment.
2. Thank your Wild Soul and Spark for gifting you such peace.

3. Over-identify with being chilled out to the point of falling over!

Mountains - When you're at the bottom of a mountain you have to climb and it feels overwhelming. Nobody can climb Everest in one giant leap, so you could...

1. Create a strong base camp by amassing all the resources you need for the ascent.
2. Break the climb into a series of small journeys and begin.
3. Just hire the best sherpa money can buy and let them sort it!

Oasis - This is where you can recover and rejuvenate when going through hard times. You could...

1. Identify what an Oasis means for you and where to find it. A spa? A massage? A loving and supportive friend you can lean on?
2. Imagine being in your inner Oasis, as in a Desert, whose palm trees shade you, fresh dates nourish you, and cool water refreshes you.
3. Decide to spend the rest of your life there and give up the struggle!

Rapids - This is where, if you've never experienced white water rafting, you'll wish you had. Turbulence, ups and downs, and a fair amount of being shaken left and right too. You could...

1. Cling on tightly knowing that, as with all life experiences, this too will pass.
2. Keeping your body soft and your eyes closed, focus deep down into your belly, nowhere to go and nothing to do, and sit for five minutes in the stillness. Repeat periodically.
3. Magic up a special Rapids' hovercraft so that you glide a few feet above whatever's going on.

River - This is when you can swim, head bobbing along, in the flow of things with no high or low emotions, just getting the job, or that aspect of life, done. You could...

1. Pat yourself on the back in congratulation for your commitment to just doing "the thang".
2. You could put treats periodically along the Riverbank to add interest.
3. Experiment with some schmoozy risk-taking to liven things up a bit.

Riverside Riveria - This is where it feels like you're in the south of France on the beach, with the sun, the sea, the sky, and the smell of great food... You could...

1. Let your body and your senses relax into the Riveria experience.
2. Collaborate with the experience by recreating Sud de la France in your home décor and lifestyle.
3. Buy a cheap bottle of plonk, a baguette, some brie and yell, "Vivre La France!"

Steep Cliffs - You feel yourself teetering on the edge of something ready to fall. This can be pleasant, even thrilling if you have a parachute, or terrifying if you haven't. You could...

1. Check whether you have a parachute or not as a priority.
2. If the latter, get one immediately even if it's metaphorical.
3. Yell "Geronimo", fling yourself over, and pray for wings!

Stuck Bog - This is where the wet decaying earth clings to your boots like sticky jam so it's virtually impossible to move. You could...

1. Take stock and look for drier patches with which to crisscross your way out of the bog.
2. Reflect on what the bog stops you from being and doing and whether that is a "good" or "not good" thing.
3. Call in helicopter backup and get yourself winched out!

Wild Flower Meadow - This is a little piece of heaven here on Earth where it's always a balmy summer's day, no toxic plants grow, and the insects don't sting. You could...

1. Drink in every nanosecond of this chill-baby-chill location.

2. Journal about your experience of it and imagine your meadow every time you need energetic nourishment.
3. Think twice if one of your Anti-life Gremlins encourages you to mow it down to ground zero!

Wilderness - This is where you wander aimlessly among boulders, scrubland, and rocky outcrops, scraping your shins and bruising your body. You could...

1. Find whatever goes by the name of a soothing stream and ease your aching body in its waters.
2. Focus on one good thing, however little, and let it be your compass to find fresh pastures.
3. Summon up Moses and ask how the hell he led his people out of there!

Woods - These can be a delight or a disturbing experience as in not seeing the wood for the trees. Be aware you are the creator of the type of Woods you experience. You could...

1. Enjoy the delightful experience, relishing the rich sun-filtering canopy and the fertile ground on which you walk.
2. Soften your gaze by using peripheral vision and ask your inner wisdom, "What am I not seeing?"
3. Call out the Teddy Bears for one helluva show-stopping picnic!

WTF Quick Sand - This is where you feel yourself being sucked into something not in your best interests or realise you have been after the event. You find yourself sinking fast. You could...

1. Call emergency services to organise your extraction like NOW. Include advice from your inner wisdom, your strategic personality part, and any other resource that will pull you out.
2. Just freakin' say NO and magic yourself away whatever the cost as your precious well-being is far more valuable.
3. Just keep saying NO and SPEAK TO THE HAND until the force of your indomitable Will catapults you to safety!

ENDNOTES

1. Beckett, S., *Waiting for Godot – A Tragicomedy in Two Acts*, 1954, New York, Grove Press.

ABOUT SHARON EDEN

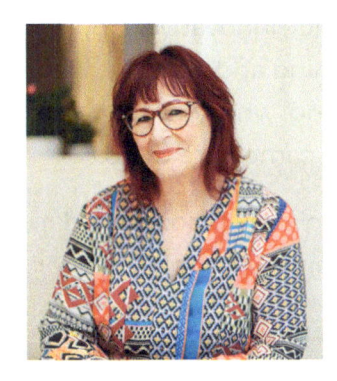

Sharon's mother had a terminal illness. A few days before she passed, Sharon was making tea in her mother's kitchen when she overheard her mother, alone in another room, say out loud, "What a waste of a life!"

Sharon was struck dumb by the impact and pain of what she heard. In the ensuing months of grief, she felt called to ensure no woman she worked with professionally would ever feel like her mother had done before she passed.

More and more women who felt discontented or lost came to work with her. They had in common a sense that something was missing and there had to be more to life but didn't know what.

Sharon realised working with these women fulfilled her calling and was her mother's legacy, as well as her own.

She is so passionate about helping as many women as possible that a book was the logical next step. So, at seventy-five, she began writing and RE-DISCOVERED was born the following year.

She knew from her history as a discontented younger woman who felt lost how the weeks could turn into years of lacklustre living, unhappiness, and even depression. She also knew it wasn't until she took action and started therapy that she and her life began to turn around.

Reading RE-DISCOVERED, with its innovative Down & Dirty Spirituality that evokes meaning and purpose, is the action needed to begin revitalising who you really are, where you're going, and what you came here to do.

As one of its endorsers said, "I absolutely bloody loved it… Makes me want to go out and hand out copies to every woman!"

Sharon Eden is a spiritual psychotherapist coach who melds ancient wisdom from the East and West with the science and art of psychotherapy and coaching in a down-to-earth way.

With over forty years of professional expertise, knowledge and wisdom, including an MA in the field, and having worked with thousands of women, she's an innovative and safe pair of hands. Sharon offers tailor-made individual programmes, master classes, and group courses.

Known as the Wild Elder, she's a woman of and connected to the Earth, the Universe, and the Divine. A woman who knows the journeys that lead you to healing, wholeness, your truth, and your own Wild Soul.

In 1965, when she was seventeen and four months pregnant, Sharon became Miss Junior South East England in a weight-lifting organisation's annual "beauty" contest. A fact that, in retrospect, causes her feminist part much angst!

You can read more about Sharon and her work, and subscribe to her free Wild Elder Weekly, at www.thewildelder.com. Access free resources mentioned in RE-DISCOVERED at www.re-discovered.life

ACKNOWLEDGEMENTS

My first is for Psychosynthesis, the psychology with soul founded by Roberto Assagioli (1888–1974) an Italian psychiatrist and pioneer of humanistic and transpersonal psychology.

Every other approach, discipline, philosophy, therapy and coaching I've learned and employ professionally rests on Psychosynthesis's impressive bedrock and is embraced by its framework.

My Down & Dirty Spirituality is entirely drawn from it.

Enormous thanks, Roberto!

Similarly, I honour those who originally trained me in Psychosynthesis, particularly Diana Whitmore and Piero Ferucci who had been Assagioli's students. And Judith Firman who helped me to embrace my juicy earthiness.

Huge loving thanks go to my beloved children, Adam Gilbert and Cassie Shoffren. They consistently give me their gorgeous support and encouragement whatever I get up to!

I feel blessed by their presence and that of their partners, Danielle and Darren, and my grandchildren, Alanna, Dayna, Naomi, Jaxon, and Zachary.

I also feel joy from the presence of Jacqueline Y B Rogers whose support and encouragement have never wavered throughout the years. And whose foreword to RE-DISCOVERED touches my heart.

Enormous freakin' thanks go to Debbie Jenkins, book coach and publisher extraordinaire, who "got" me and my voice. And to everyone on her team, including Lisa de Caux for her sensitive editing and Jayr Cuario for making RE-DISCOVERED look so gorgeous.

Not forgetting my amazing book-writing cohort peers, Anne Walsh and David Pullan.

With Debbie at our helm, we've laughed hysterically together, supported and encouraged one another, and taken the mick out of each other gloriously, especially out of David! I'll miss our regular meetings.

Huge thanks to my Beta readers, Jacqueline Y B Rogers, Rachel Levy, Bernie Edwards and Cassie Shoffren, for their feedback in all its glory and my brand photographer Brigitta Schloz-Mastroianni who captures my Wild Soul every time.

Similar huge thanks to all the awesome people who've endorsed REDISCOVERED and whose names light up its pages.

And, finally, to the thousands of magnificent women I've worked with individually or in groups, in person or online, my heartfelt thanks for the privilege and the learning.

To coin a phrase, live long and prosper, precious ones...

MORE PRAISE FOR RE-DISCOVERED

Adventure with Sharon through the pits of fear and the bogs of stuckness to discover you can climb to new heights, making friends with the deep joy that has always lived inside you. Let this Wild Elder lead you on an easy-to-follow, real-life mystical quest into the YOU ready to emerge from your chrysalis.

Soleira Green, Visionary Author,
Future Innovator, Quantum Coach, and
Author of 17 books including "The New Visionaries:
Evolutionary Leadership for a Vibrant World"

RE-DISCOVERED is a must-read for every woman who is interested in self-development or who has gone through adversity. This book is for you if you're dipping your toe or are fully in the know about spirituality. Buy it, read it, LIVE it!

Amanda FitzGerald,
Multi Award Winning PR & Visibility Strategist

I absolutely bloody love it. It was powerful, raw, honest, warm, and funny. It resonated, it got me thinking, it made me laugh out loud, shout yessss (and nooo!) and get a moist eye. I'm going to re-read it, again and again.

An achingly honest, down-to-earth, eye-opening page-turner that WILL get you thinking. Makes me want to go outside and hand copies out to every woman I see. No ifs, buts or maybes, just bloody read it.

Rachel Levy, The Marketing Hive,
Multi Award Winning Marketing Support

If you have ever felt there is a missing piece, or even missing peace, in your life, then RE-DISCOVERED can help you to literally reconnect with your uniquely valuable resources and bring them from dormant to vibrant life.

Christine Miller, MA, FRSA

As a scientist, I have had a weird relationship with spirituality, but Sharon's honest, sometimes laugh-out-loud words have helped me make sense of some parts of my life and be absolutely OK with bits that don't make sense. RE-DISCOVERED is a fabulous resource for compassionately understanding yourself at a deep level.

Gill McKay, Award Winning Speaker and Educator
about alcohol harm in life and work, Author of "Stuck:
Brain Smart Insights for Coaches"

Told from a self-experienced perspective, there is everything to help us through today's troubles to tomorrow's growth. This is a desk/bedside reference must-have.

Sheila Hinchliffe,
80 year old, Pagan, retired Computer Analyst

More Praise For Re-Discovered

RE-DISCOVERED is a treasure trove of Sharon's wisdom and expertise intertwined with her inspiring story that takes you on a delicious journey to connect with and unleash your Wild Soul and take on becoming the woman you deserve to be in line with your true self.

Kate Porter, The Midlife Metamorphosis Coach and Founder of Second Spring Life Coaching

Reading RE-DISCOVERED is like getting a delightful spiritual jolt—Sharon's wit and wisdom guide you through self-discovery with a smile. It's the most fun I've had while unravelling the mysteries of my very wild soul!

Debbie Jenkins, Author & Publisher

"Down & Dirty Spirituality" takes on the life issue you thought you could ignore; isn't there more to life than this? Leave RE-DISCOVERED alone unless you want to take on Eden's straight-talking and use its tools to get to the heart of why you and your spirituality matter and what you can do about it.

Dr Phyllis SantaMaria,
Co-Founder of the Award Winning "Social Impact Game"

RE-DISCOVERED's practical grounded and inclusive approach to spiritual growth has given me the tools to better support my clients' wellbeing. It is an invitation to embark on a path of introspection, discovery, and empowerment.

Susannah Simmons, The Feel Good Fitness Coach

If you are a woman of a certain age who is feeling lost and asking herself, "Is this it?" this book is for you. A book to be re-discovered many times chock-a-block full of compassion and hope.

Anne Walsh, The Excel Lady, Author of "HATE EXCEL"

To have this positive, purposeful and enlightening book to hand to reflect on how to best navigate the diverse complexities of our own lives and, consequently, to feel we are not alone in this, is a very powerful and much-needed resource.

Sarah Szekir-Papasavva,
Multi Award Winning Virtual Assistant,
Apt Virtual Assistance Ltd

Sharon's deliciously wicked sense of humour paired with her obvious care for other human beings made me feel seen, heard and understood, like a gigantic hug with a side of encouragement. The deeper spiritual work expertly guides you through practices that enlighten you without ever creating pressure for a particular outcome.

Joanne Fazel,
Initial Teacher Training Administrator, Teach West London

An inspiring read! Part biography, part novel, part psychology classes made easy and a whole load of therapy sessions all in one. A few tears and lots of laughs, I was gripped till the end. I will be re-reading RE-DISCOVERED over and over again.

Nadia Abdul,
Founder of Change Maker Inc.